Ix Hmer ...ya
Maya Herbal Medicine

The Creator created humans and they started to wonder if they were alone on earth and if they had the power and knowledge they needed to survive on earth. They said we are weak and don't have power, so the jaguar came and said. "I will give you my power and strength." They said, "What will I do when I get sick?" And the snake came and said, "I will give you the knowledge of the plants." And that is how we got the knowledge of the plants.

There was a lady who wanted to learn about the plants, the knowledge about herbal medicine, sewing, embroidery, and measuring. We now know this lady as Ix Chel, the goddess of medicine and childbirth.

She consulted an elder who recommended that she had to get ready for that, to fast and do ceremonies for several days until she was ready to get the knowledge. When the elder thought that she was ready, they took her to the nest of the leaf-cutter ants. She had to dance around the hole nine times, clockwise and counter-clockwise, singing and doing all the enchantments. She was told that when she did that, the father of the serpents would emerge from that hole.

That serpent, when it appears, it would be the Och Can, the one that doesn't bite, the boa constrictor. She would be licked all over her body from head to toe by this snake. Then he would lie down on the ground. Then she was told to copy the patterns on the skin of the boa constrictor and other snakes by embroidering counted needlethread (*xoc' bi chui'*). That is where she got the knowledge of healing, weaving, embroidery, sewing, and any architectual or other measuring. She took the power of the midwifry, sewing, healing, and measuring. That is how we believe it came to happen.

This legend was told to me by my mother who heard it from her father.
— Aurora Garcia Saqui

Dedication

I dedicate this book in memory of my great-uncle, Don Elijio Panti, who was known at the time of his death as one of the greatest healers in Belize and Central America. He was born in El Peten, Guatemala, and came to Succotz, Cayo, the village near Xunantunich. After he got married to my grandmother's sister, he moved to my village. There he started to heal at the age of 34 years. As I was growing up, he was the only healer in my village. Family members believe that he was 110 years old at the time of his death, but it could not be verified because he had no records of his birth. He was buried with honors, arranged by the government of Belize with the Belizean flag wrapped around his coffin. The Belize Defence Force gave the last salute. He was known as one of the remnants of the ancient Maya left behind because he didn't know the value of money.

Don Elijio represents the past. I also want to dedicate this book to the children of Belize, our future, that they might gain this knowledge and learn to respect the plants and see their value.

— Aurora Garcia Saqui
August, 2015

Other Books by Aurora Garcia Saqui

U Janal Aj Maya: Traditional Mayan Cuisine by Aurora Garcia Saqui with Amy Lichty, 2013. Caye Caulker, Belize: *Producciones de la Hamaca.*

H'men Herb Center and Botanical Garden by Aurora Garcia Saqui with photographs by Eric A. Kessler, 2003.

Ix Hmen U Tzaco Ah Maya:
Maya Herbal Medicine

Aurora Garcia Saqui

**Dorothy Beveridge and
Judy Lumb, Editors**

Producciones de la Hamaca
Caye Caulker, BELIZE

Photos by Judy Lumb and Dorothy Beveridge

Published by *Producciones de la Hamaca*
Caye Caulker, BELIZE
<producciones-hamaca.com>

ISBN: 978-976-8142-86-3 (print edition)
ISBN: 978-976-8142-87-0 (e-book edition)

Front Cover*:* Painting of the Mayan Goddess Ix Chel by Aurora Garcia Saqui, who explains, "We believe that the moon is feminine and the person that appears as one gazes at the full moon is Ix Chel, the Mayan goddess of healing. She is also the goddess of the moon, but we are not allowed to gaze at the moon. We were taught as children not to stare at the moon because we revere Ix Chel so much. Staring at someone is very disrespectful. We can glance, but not stare." This is a book about Mayan traditional healing, so Ix Chel in the moon occupies the front cover.

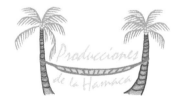

Producciones de la Hamaca is dedicated to:
- Celebration and documentation of Belize's rich, diverse cultural heritage,
- Protection and sustainable use of Belize's remarkable natural resources,
- Inspired, creative expression of Belize's spiritual depth.

Table of Contents

Acknowledgements vi
Introduction 1
Traditional Maya Herbal Medicine 9
  Collecting Medicinal Plants 9
  Baths 10
  Acupuncture 11
  Copal Sacred Incense 12
  Cough Syrup 12
  Cupping 12
  Gel 13
  Good Luck Charms 14
  Insect Repellent 15
  Oil 15
  Oil for Massage 15
  Ointment 15
  Poultice 16
  Powder 16
  Prayers 16
  Smudge 17
  Tea 18
  Tincture 18
  Tonic 18

Remedies for Common Illnesses and Complaints 19
   AIDS 19
   Allergies 19
   Anemia 19
   Anger 20
   Arthritis and Rheumatism 20
   Asthma 20
   Athlete's Foot 20
   Bad Spirits and Bad Luck 21
   Balance 21
   Beef Worm 21
   Behaviour Problems 21
   Bleeding 21
   Blood Pressure 22
   Blood Purifier 22
   Breast-feeding 22
   Burns 23
   Cancer 23
   Cold, Cough, and Flu 24
   Contraception 24
   Dehydration 25
   Depression 25
   Diabetes 26
   Digestion Problems 26
   Ears 27
   Evil Eyes 27
   Eyes 27
   Fever 28
   General Health 28
   Hair 29
   Headache and Migraine 29
   Hepatitis 30
   Immune System 30

Infertility 30

Inflammation 30

Laxative 30

Menopause Hot Flashes 31

Menstruation 31

Mumps 31

Muscle Weakness and Paralysis 31

Muscle Cramps 31

Pain 31

Pregnancy and Delivery 31

Protection 32

Purge 32

Skin Lesions 32

Sleep Problems 33

Sore Throat and Tonsillitis 34

Snakebite 34

Sprains 34

Stomach Ulcers 34

Stress 34

Stroke (Mild) 34

Thorn 35

Tobacco Smoking Addiction 35

Toothache.. 35

Trauma... 35

Tumor (non-malignant) 35

Urinary Problems 35

Vision 36

Weight Reduction 36

Worms 36

Wound Healing 37

Herbal Plant Identification................................ 38

My Hopes for the Future 154

References 156

Index 157

Acknowledgements

I would like to thank all the people who have contributed to the production of this book. Thanks to Emily Carlson, Julie Wright, students who interned with me in order to learn about Mayan culture and traditional healing, and assisted in the preservation of our cultural knowledge helping with this and other books. Also thank you to Creation Care Studies Program and Pro Belize, programmes who have helped my dreams come true through connecting me with my interns. It is great that we have programmes like these in Belize.

I would like to thank Judy Lumb and Dorothy Beveridge for helping me and having the interest to publish this book. Dorothy used her environmental experience to search high and low to find the scientific names for most of the plants I use. She used her creativity to design the book. Judy came to spend time with us and worked hard taking the photos and put on her boots to go into the forest with me to make sure all of this is documented. I feel blessed for having all these good people around me.

I am especially grateful to my great-uncle, Elijio Panti, the well-known Mayan healer who shared his knowledge with me. Thanks also to my grandfather, Juan Pascal Mesh, my grand-mother, Onoria Mesh, and my mother and father, Aureliano and Paulina Garcia for passing on their knowledge. Special thanks to my sisters, Maria, Carmelita, Silvia, Paulita, and my brother Heraldo (Marroquin) for always being beside me. Thanks to Ernesto for being a supportive and loving husband. Thanks to my children, Rigoberto, Gabriel, and Marroquin.

I want to thank everybody from San Antonio, Cayo, my village place of birth where everybody still speaks Maya. May God keep blessing each and everyone, that they may have strength to keep passing all the knowledge to our children because it is very important. Let us keep the example of our grandparents.

With all my heart
Aurora G. Saqui, J.P.

Dios Botik ti tulacal maco San Antonio in Cahal, kin wiyic hach maloob ichil in puzical in gatesh hash yaba kin zibtic E lela Ete tulaca in wool, kin woyik minan u lak cah bis Eh Tanah tush tulacaloon kic tanic ich Maya. Dios ku yilooon ete mas muuc yoko ku pahtale ik mansic Tulaca ik wohe ti Eh palaloobo. Bis u metaho ik nolo Dios Botic. Ti in tio Don Elijio Panti u mansa ten tulacal u yolo. Mu pah ta Lin tuubsikesh. Dios Botic.

Ete tulacal in wool
Aurora G. Saqui, J.P.

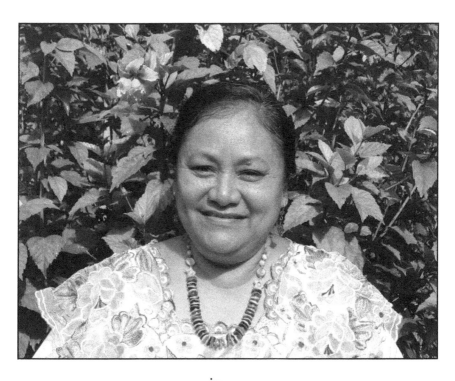

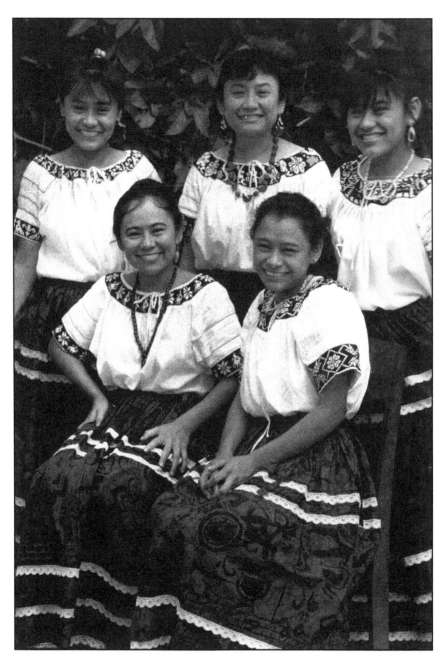

Garcia Sisters in the 1980s
(*back row, from left*) Aurora, Maria, Sylvia
(*front row, from left*) Piedad, Carmelita

Introduction

Iwas born Aurora Aureliana Garcia on the 13th of June in 1967, a birthday I share with the patron saint of my village, San Antonio, Cayo, Belize. I grew up on the family farm, Abolito. My father, Aureliano Garcia, came to San Antonio from the village of Bullet Tree in the northwest of Belize. There he met my mother Paulina Mesh and had six children: Maria, Heraldo Marroquin, Piedad, Aurora, Carmelita, and Silvia.

As we were growing up, my siblings and I heard legends of the gods and stories important to Maya culture. I never thought my family was special in any way and certainly never believed that my work would involve using knowledge that I gained as a young child, knowledge that is of such importance to my culture and country. However, with the benefit of hindsight I now believe that my sisters and I were given the gift of art by the god, Pauatun, who was often depicted in images around our home. According to Maya legends, if a god is shown to you often, it is a message that you have been given a gift of extraordinary talent. This gift was granted to us by the Alux (Tata Duende) who is the representative of Pauatun.

In this case, my sisters and I were given the gift of art and have become famous for our beautiful slate carvings. It all began when I was put to work on the farm along with my siblings. In 1981 whilst tilling the earth in a peanut field, we discovered a black stone that we had not seen before. Taking it home, we began to use the stone as a part of our artwork. It happened that at the same time of the slate discovery, an excavation of a Maya site was taking place nearby. One of the archaeologists residing with our family commented that if we depicted the images of Mayan gods and other legends on the slate, they could sell them and this could become a vital tool in preserving the ancient Maya culture. Until that day, I had never realized that my people were a unique civilization.

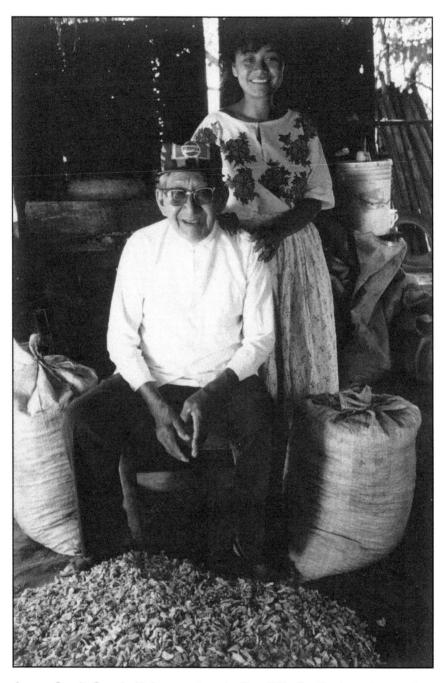

Aurora Garcia Saqui with her great-uncle, Don Elijio Panti, when she was in her teens. They are surrounded by bags of herbs that have been chopped, dried, and then bagged until needed for healing.

Shortly after this encounter, my sisters and I set about building our own business to sell our product. In addition to the slate carvings, we displayed other pieces of art, jewelry and historical artifacts. As time passed, our fame grew and so did the demand for our artwork. We received large orders, were featured in newspapers, and became a tourist attraction in Belize. The slate-carvings were an eye-opening that made us look at how important our culture is, and what can we do to preserve it. From there we dedicated ourselves to preserve what we have left and to tell others to pass the knowledge on so that it can continue.

At the age of sixteen, I approached my great-uncle, the famous herbal healer, Don Elijio Panti, and asked if he would teach me about all the herbs. I only wanted to preserve his knowledge for future generations, but not to do his work. I know that deep in his heart he wanted me not only to have it for myself, but to publish for the world. In doing this book, his legend continues. I hope all who use this information, will do it in memory of him.

My uncle was very happy to take me on as his apprentice, so I accompanied Panti every morning from six until eight on his daily trips to the jungle for many years. He told me that going early was the best time to pick herbs as they would be fresher and the medicinal aspects of the plant would be of better quality.

I asked him how many of the plants around us were medicine and he said, "Everything, except you have to learn how to use them."

He emphasized the importance of respecting all these different things because they have an owner. We have to pay for what we take because it is not for us, it is for them. We have to ask permission, so whatever herb he collected, he asked that plant for permission. He taught me to do ceremonies through the year. Once a year he did a thanksgiving ceremony.

When Panti told me that after he died I would be the one to take over his position as herbal healer, I replied that I could not, as I was too busy with my artwork. He laughed at me in a way that he knew what the future would bring even if I did not. In Mayan culture one cannot do another's work until after they have died, even if you have trained under him.

At the age of twenty-four I married Ernesto Saqui, Cockscomb Basin Wildlife Sanctuary Park Director, and moved to the village of Maya Centre in the Stann Creek District. At this time my uncle was

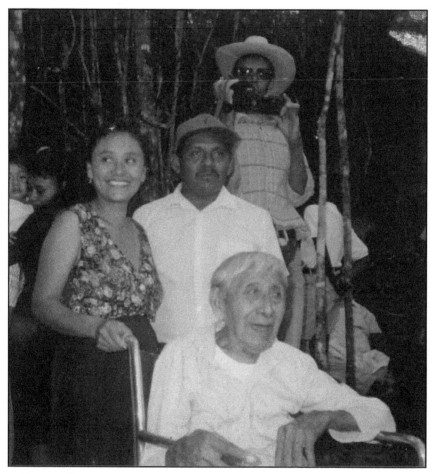

Aurora Garcia Saqui, with her husband Ernesto Saqui, wheeling her elderly great-uncle Don Elijio Panti in 1993, eight years before he died.

beginning to become very weak. He gave me a bag, inside of which I found his crystals, jade stones, glasses for cupping, and sting ray spines to use for acupuncture. He asked me if I had found my own crystal after the sacrifice I made to the gods to bring me the gift of healing. At first I said that I had not, but at that moment realized that in fact I had found it, but failed to recognize it. On an excursion into the forest with my father we stopped at a river. On the river bed floor I spotted a shiny marble, but presuming that it had been left by a child I did not pick

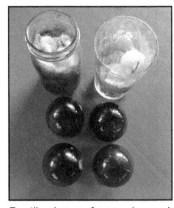

Panti's glasses for cupping and crytals given to Aurora

it up. My uncle told me that this was my gift from the gods as they had put it in my path for me to find it.

About a month later at my home in Maya Centre I had a dream that my uncle was calling my name so loudly and clearly that I believed he was really there. "Mama (his name for me), get up! It is your time to heal the people!" He also mentioned a particular herb, the yax le'e. Panti had often described this herb as the father of all the healings that is used as an ingredient in many medicines.

Later that morning a young man about the age of 17 came to me for help. He had a severe case of arthritis and could barely walk. To help him I made a special medicine for arthritis using the very same herb that my uncle spoke of in my dream. That began my work as a healer. A little later that day I received a telephone call from my sister in San Antonio saying that my uncle had died that morning around six o'clock.

From that day forward I have had hundreds of people come to me for help. Every day people come from all over Belize to ask my

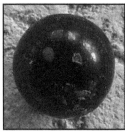

advice and receive treatment, and their numbers are ever increasing. A few weeks after the death of my uncle, the creek in Maya Centre flooded. I went down to the banks of the creek after it had gone down and was back to its regular clear water. Whilst sifting through the stones and pebbles I caught sight of something. It was a gift from the gods, my crystal, and this time I picked it up.

Crystal Aurora found

The healing that I do is different from what a doctor does because I take a spiritual approach. People come to me when they have been to doctors and the problem was not solved. In a few cases amputations were recommended by the doctor, but when they got herbs from me, they got better, and did not have to go through with the amputation.

Most of my patients want a reading with a crystal. That is where I start. It tells me what type of energy they have, what is their real problem. We believe that when we go around people we pick up their energies. If you go around people with bad energy, you can get contaminated. It can give a bad spell, *mal de ojo*, the evil eye, which can make you get sick, or it can give you a lot of bad luck, getting into accidents, losing your things, money comes and goes like water. Those are the symptoms.

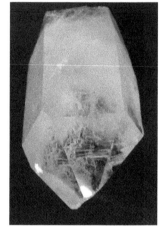

crystal

I use the crystal for a lot of things; I can make predictions with it. If a family member is lost, they want to know where they are, if they are alive. A girl got lost when they went fishing. She went back for a gallon of water, but she was walking last, so no one noticed that she had turned back. They waited and waited and she didn't come. The whole village went looking until dark. Then the next morning the mother came to me and wanted to know if she was alive or if animals got her. I went to my crystal. I could see the girl running toward the sea, so I knew she was OK. She was just lost, running the wrong way. She came back that morning. She finally got to the highway and a truck brought her home.

In some cases my patients need only the prayers. These prayers are not now-a-day prayers, they are recited in Maya. They are not invoking God or bad spirits. I invoke my patient; the prayers are recited to the pulse or muscles. This is also done with babies. As a Maya person, we grow up with this. If a baby cries in their sleep, that means he is frightened. By touching the pulses and the head while reciting a special prayer, the baby is balanced, calmed, and can go back to sleep. The next time he goes to sleep, he won't cry in his sleep again.

If this is not corrected, that same symptom can develop a heart problem, even as an adult. It might start to appear as a nervous system problem, mild fever, upset stomach, diarrhea, high or low blood pressure, chronic indigestion, or depression. All these can develop from one problem, imbalance of energies.

After I have seen the energies in the crystal, if they have a physical problem, then I heal them with herbs. One herb can be used for several problems. For example, guava bark can be used for diarrhea, but also heals cuts or wounds, and helps the womb heal after giving birth. Suppose a person has depression, we would give them some herbs to bathe at home. Besides taking a bath, I would also recommend smudging with smoke, and cleansing spiritually outside. I would brush the patient with a piece of shrub to take away the negativity and throw it in the river so it goes away. Then I would give him herbs to make tea to drink.

Sometimes I dream remedies. I had a stone in my gall bladder, that was first diagnosed when I was pregnant, but the doctor didn't recommend doing anything about it because I was pregnant. Five years later I was awakened by a sharp pain. I was dreaming that someone was bringing something for me. He had a stem and fruit of the plant, mosote, in the palm of his hand. He said to use the stem, but he brought the fruit so I could recognize the plant. When I woke up I went looking for the plant, but I couldn't find it. Then I was doing my wash and it was right there. I put the stems in the palm of my hand like it was in my dream. As soon as the stem hit my hand, I knew what to do and thought, "why is it that we don't know how to heal ourselves?" The plant talked to me and I knew that is what I needed to take for my problem. I took it every day for a week and the pain was gone. I still take it now and again, and the ultrasound shows that I have no gall stones.

Plant remedies do not have to be from exotic, far-away places. Often the herb you need is right in front of you, the most common plant. This happened to me when I was having problems with my womb. I discovered that hog plum bark tea, trees that are everywhere around, completely solved the problem with my womb.

We, the Maya, are a community of people who still trust in herbal medicines. The reason for writing this book is to preserve some of our Mayan knowledge because very few people are documenting the knowledge of herbal medicines today, especially the herbalists themselves. Though I am young, I am afraid that the recognized value of plants and their medicinal purposes will be lost if not written down before I die. I am very fortunate to have learned from my great-uncle, Elijio Panti, and I believe it is part of my responsibility to pass this knowledge to both older and younger generations.

I want to encourage young people to become healers. In preparing to be a healer, it is easier to start when you are young, innocent, and pure. Your consciousness is clean and you learn faster. To become a healer, you must not think about the money part of it. Instead you have to think about helping people. While learning, you have to fast sometimes. You have to have great respect for the spiritual beings that care for the plants, the mountains, and the water.

I write to encourage other herbalists to sustain their practices with traditional medicines. I urge you, readers and herbalists, through your understanding of Mayan culture and traditional healing to teach your children or somebody close to you what you know. I say this in hope that the knowledge will be kept alive for future generations just as our ancestors have done for us, especially for all Belizeans. I give these recipes for all who can use them with all my heart.

My hope is that Belizeans continue to appreciate what we have in our country that is so rich in its vast plant life. I hope this appreciation will bring about a preservation of the forest and the plants that ancient Mayan cultures have used for thousands of years.

In the next chapter I describe the methods I use for preparing herbs for healing. Then I give my favorite recipes for how I combine the herbs that I give patients for particular illnesses and complaints. In the chapter on herbal plant identification, I have provided photos, along with some identifying features, and the purposes of each plant with hopes that you may be able to identify some of them in the wild and use them for remedies in your home.

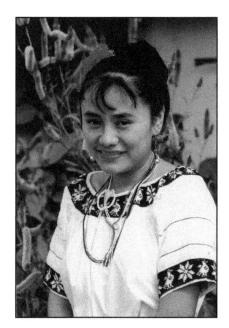

Aurora Garcia
as a young woman

Traditional Mayan Herbal Medicine

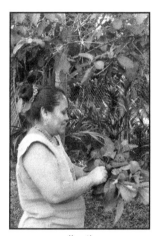
collecting

For thousands of years, our great ancestors have been using Mayan herbal medicines, which have survived through the generations. Mayan medicines are known to have few side effects. The following are the methods I use for healing and preparing herbal remedies. Other healers may use other herbs, other methods, or the same herbs for different ailments.

Collecting Medicinal Plants

Part of collecting herbs is that you have to give thanks. We don't call them gods, but there are spiritual beings that care for the plants, animals, waterways, lagoons, mountains, roads and everything else in the forest. We respect them so much that we are afraid of them. We don't want to offend them, because that is when a bad spell may come, bad luck or anything that is hurtful. My uncle showed me the special prayers to connect with those spiritual beings. We have to offer something in reward for what we are using. We do special porridge with corn or we can offer incense, too.

When I connect with the spiritual beings of the plants, they communicate with me, not talking, but when I go to the jungle I feel the connection, which plants are good for healing and which ones I have to be careful of. The connection with the plants also comes in my dreams. When I have a patient with a new sickness that I don't know what plant to use, I dream about a plant, use it, and they get healed.

Plants can be collected any time, but it is better to collect in the mornings because the plants have dew and are fresh. When collecting I have to ask them to help me heal the person. I tell the plant, "You are put on earth to help humans. Help us and heal us." I usually talk to the plants in Yucatec Maya. *"U tza'hecho ti jaanta yoc'ol cab. Ka' waanteen y ka tzäkeen."*

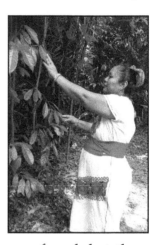

Baths

Holistic herbal baths are used to activate all the good energies and wash away the bad energies. For holistic baths, pipers are preferred, but there must be nine species because nine is the sacred number, so other plants could be added if there are not nine piper species. Baths can also be used for nervousness, depression, anxiety, and stress. If the bath is for healing, alepa, madre cacao, pheasant tail, rudah, basil, pipers, and ix tuc'ulil are added for a total of nine species. Collect a handful of leaves of each of nine species. Smash the leaves and soak them for a few hours in a bucket of water and bathe with it, washing everything from head to toe. Put it in the sun for an hour or two to warm it, or take the bath at natural temperature. Scrub yourself with the leaves of the herbs in the water. Use all the water and do not rinse, but leave it to dry. When finished, collect all the leaves and push them under a dead tree that has dropped, or throw it into the river or the sea to get rid of bad energy.

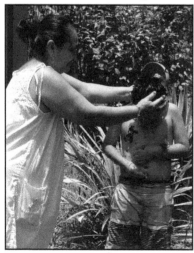

pouring

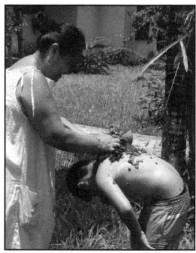

scrubbing

A hot bath can be used for "pasmo," which is when your blood is getting too thick. This occurs with a sudden change in temperature, like getting wet in the rain when working hard in the fields. This can cause a high fever. When my uncle tried acupuncture in a case like this, no blood would come out because it was too thick. "Pasmo" is also the name of a plant. Boil a handful of leaves of pasmo; any citrus, such as, lime, orange or sour orange; plus avocado, wild oregano, and piper leaves with the juice of one lime in two to three liters of water for about ten minutes. Add more water to cool it just enough so you can stand it and pour it over yourself in a closed room. Stay in a closed room for a day and a half after you bathe. You should avoid fan, air-conditioning, or wind, especially wind of rain, for another day and a half or you can get sicker.

Acupuncture

Called "*pirish*" in Maya, "*pik*" in Creole, or "*punse*" in Spanish, acupuncture is used because some bad blood has to be let out. We believe that there is some toxin that needs to be released. It is used for problems like facial paralysis, membrane headaches, or pains in different parts of the body. We never use metal for acupuncture, because metal tools have "*ki'nam*," which means more pain or more infection. Instead we use thorns from palms, cockspur, ceiba, or citrus trees; porcupine quills, stingray spines, or shards of glass. After puncturing, cupping is often used to suck out the tension or pain.

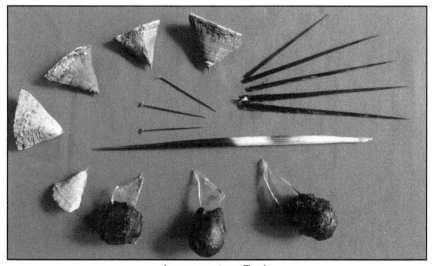

Accupuncture Tools
In the outer circle at the bottom are three broken pieces of glass embedded in black beeswax; around the circle to the left are five Ceiba thorns; to the right are five thorns from the Cocoyol or Supa Palm; inside are three thorns from Wari Palm and a porcupine quill.

Copal Sacred Incense

During the dry season, cut straight lines in the copal tree (*pom*) with a container underneath to catch the falling resin. Leave it for a few days to collect the resin. To burn, make charcoal, and put the incense on the coal for a lot of smoke. When burned, the incense purifies the air. It chases away evil spirits and brings peace to your life. When you burn incense, you are feeding or revering the gods. There are lots of reasons for making the offering: you may want to cleanse your house of evil spirits; you may want to ask permission to go to hunt or to clear a plantation; you may want to bless a new relationship in a wedding. If you are burning copal as an offering, choose a special place (mountains, caves, modern or ancient temples, tops of hills, higher elevations), a place where you can get a better connection. Then burn only the copal without charcoal. Use a little pine to light it and offer at least one pound of copal.

For cleansing or purification of a house, burn the incense only on sacred Mayan days: Tuesdays, Thursdays, or Fridays in the evenings (between six pm and twelve midnight). Offerings for the gods or for special occasions such as weddings can be done on any day. For purification of a house, burn the copal with anise seed and rosemary leaves. If you want to chase evil spirits out of a house, burn the copal with garlic and tobacco in the evening. If you want to bring good luck and peace in a house with too much fighting or children rebelling, burn copal with a pinch of sage, sugar or honey, cinnamon, tobacco, and garlic in the evening. For birthdays, christening, burials, and weddings, burn only copal on charcoal without any herbs.

Cough Syrup

Crush a handful of leaves from cotton, young mango, avocado, soursop, lemongrass, thick oregano, and verbena. Boil in one liter of water for 15 minutes and strain it. Add one pound of sugar. Put it to boil until it thickens, maybe 30 minutes more. Refrigerate and it will last for six months.

Cupping

Most of the time acupuncture is used with cupping, a form of massage using a glass with fire inside that is applied on the skin. A

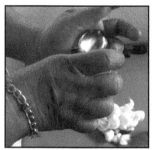 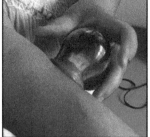 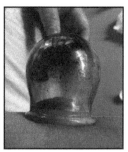

Cupping: light cotton   place glass upside down   suction

small piece of copal or chewing gum is stuck on the side of a small drinking glass. A piece of cotton is stuck to the copal or chewing gum, lit, and the glass put upside down on the skin. As the fire goes out, it creates suction. The glass is then moved around on the skin, maintaining the suction. A larger glass can be used for larger areas of the body. It is very effective for back pain. Acupuncture can be applied first and then use cupping to pull the blood out. This removes toxins and is good for paralysis.

Gel

Gels are for topical application, usually for pain, such as for sports injuries, arthritis, or headaches. To make the gel, boil a half pound of seaweed in one liter of water for ten to fifteen minutes until it is dissolved, or use commercial "Ice Gel." Let it cool so it will gel. Grind the herbs and add a small amount of water to the ground herbs to add to the gel. Add one cup of rum or rubbing alcohol for every liter of water to preserve the gel. Mix and use topically.

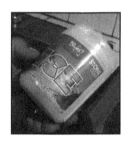

Commercial
Ice Gel

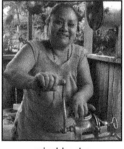 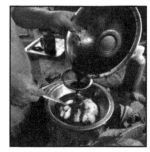 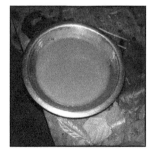

grind herbs   add herbs to gel   prepared gel

Good Luck Charms

There are three types of good luck charms (*qui cun naj*). The red one is for love, the black one protects you from everything negative, and the green one protects your belongings and money against misfortune and evil spells. It is good for businesses, too.

Mayan good luck charms use sacred plants: anise seed, copal, lavender flowers, rosemary and sage leaves. The leaves must be dried. For the green one I add rice, cacao seed, and corn. I use new, small red, black, or green cloth to sew a pillow for them. It is very important that the cloth be new.

A prayer must be said with the crystal ball in the name of the person who is going to use it. I use several crystals in a circle around the good luck charm to activate it. If it is for love, for protection, or for belongings, I enchant it for that particular energy. It blocks the person from the negative energies and gives them good luck.

Any object can be activated as a good luck charm: plants, rocks, dust, chalk, or metal, preferably silver or gold. The charm is to be carried with you wherever you go.

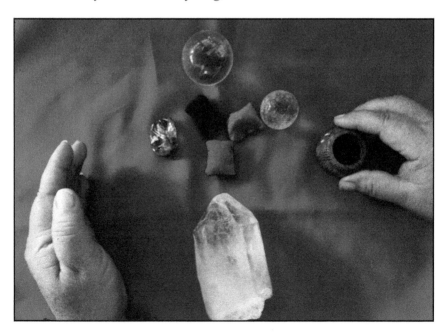

Aurora Saqui is energizing three good luck charms for a patient. Three pouches filled with sacred herbs are shown: green for prosperity, black for protection, and red for love.

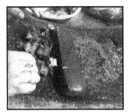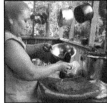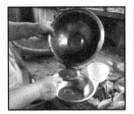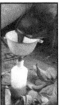

making insect repellant from fresh herbs

Insect Repellent

This remedy is both a repellent and an anti-itch tincture for mosquito and other insect bites. Make the tincture from beneno xut, ko'mo' che', jackass bitters, gumbolimbo, a few leaves of pipers, and polly redhead.

Oil

Cohune oil is obtained by grinding kernels into small pieces and boiling for a few hours while the oil rises to the surface. It is then skimmed off the water surface and refried until dry.

Oil for Massage

For massage oil, holistic plants are used, including pipers, madre cacao, rudah, basil, sage, and ma'mu'kal. Collect these plants and make this oil on the full moon because then the moon has its full power. All the plants are energized by the full moon, so they are stronger in their properties. Grind the leaves together. Fry a handful of the ground herbs in any oil: coconut, cohune, olive, or cooking oil. Add the fried herbs to one liter of oil. This massage oil gives good energy, keeps you going, and makes your immune system strong so you don't get sick. I use this oil every day when I go to work because I see a lot of sick people and this protects me from getting sick.

Ointment

Ointments (*bok*) are used topically for skin problems, such as sores, cuts, rashes, and insect bites. Grind a handful of a combination of leaves and add to one cup of pork fat and half a pound of bee's wax. Cook under low heat for about ten minutes. Strain before it hardens in a metal sieve that can stand the heat. Place in a jar with a big opening.

Poultice

A poultice is an application of fresh herbs for bruises, inflammation, infections, insect or snake bites to draw out the toxins and cool
off the infection or inflammation. Macerate as many different piper
leaves as you have, plus coffee or cacao powder, and one egg, blend
it all together, place on the affected area, and tie it with a piece
of cloth so it will not drop. Powder already prepared can also be
used. Add just enough water, rubbing alcohol, or brandy to wet the
mixture. A poultice can be applied to the palm of the hand, bottom
of the foot, or over the belly for patients that are so sick that they
cannot eat.

Powder

Powder can be used instead of liquid because it is easier to carry.
Powder is also good to store plants for as long as a year if well
sealed. Use leaves, soft stems, or bark. Dry leaves or stems in the
sun and grind them to make a powder. Grind bark without drying
it first. To take internally, just put a bit on your tongue. On the skin
sprinkle the powder on the injury. Powder is very effective for serious wounds that you cannot wet because they are too infected, or
rotten like gangrene, such as those that have already been recommended for amputation.

Prayers

Prayers are important for healing. There are different prayers for
different health issues and one prayer that is recommended for
everyone, even if they are not sick. That type of healing is called in
Spanish "*ensalmo*," in Maya, "*patz*." This particular healing is good
for balance, blood flow, heartbeat, chronic fever, blood pressure,
nervous system, and digestive system, trauma, and cleanses the
aura.

The prayers are passed down through the generations. Healers are
respected because they keep the prayers that ordinary people do
not know. We use prayers because we believe that in order to heal
someone, the healer must connect with the spiritual being of the
patient. The healer begins by holding the right hand of the person
palm up. The right hand is where you receive the connection. I
recite prayers while pressing the pulse with a leaf of a sacred herb
or black beeswax from wild bees. The patient receives it through
the palm of the hand. Then prayers are recited on the left wrist,
and the forehead, making an upside-down "V" shape. That shape

is used because the healer wants the person to recover, so it points up toward the heavenly powers so that person can overcome whatever he is going through. Either pipers or pheasant tail can be used. This absorbs all the negative energy to be banished with the setting of the sun or to be washed away by the river. Then throw the herbs away with your left hand at a crossroad by turning your back toward the sunset and throw it back over your head. Don't look back, only forward. Or you can throw the leaves in the river with your back to the river or the sea. Again, don't look backward, but continue forward. You can bury it where you will not pass too often or put it under dead log.

For whole body spiritual cleansing, you can use a branch of any of these: frijolillo, any piper, pheasant tail, wild berry, or malva. Wet the branch with white rum (*baalche ha'*) and pass it over the person from the head down, front and back, while saying the person's name and reciting a prayer. Then throw the branch as described above.

It is best to throw the herbs used for spiritual cleansing at sunset. The herbs can be sealed in a black plastic bag. Keep it away from you until you can throw it away. We believe that as the sun goes down, it carries away all the negativity because there is nothing that is more powerful than the sun.

Smudge

Mix a piece of copal about an inch square with a pinch of anise seed, rosemary, frankincense, tobacco, and a clove of garlic. Burn it three, seven, or nine times. Put the mixture on a hot coal and put it in a dish. Never use an incense burner because we believe if you use an incense burner you are inviting death or bad luck for the person. If you want a companion or peace in your home, you can combine cinnamon, sage, rice, coffee, and sugar, or at least cinnamon and sugar. If you want to call for food, add rice, cacao, and coffee. You can smudge your house by burning in the middle of the house.

Or, you can smudge yourself. It is best to be alone because if anyone else is there, that person might get contaminated by the bad energy leaving you. In a closed up room, sit on a chair and put the container with the smoke under the chair. Cover yourself with a sheet. Expel whatever negativity you want to remove by saying it nine times out loud. Then call for whatever you want nine times. For example, if you want a companion, you will say, "Love come to me" nine times.

Take all the smoke until it burns out. Do this in the evening and then rest. Do not go outside. The next day get rid of the sheet by burning or burying it. Put on clean clothes and either wash the clothes and rinse in lime or vinegar, or, if you are trying to get rid of bad spirits, burn or bury the clothes.

Tea

Tea is the most common way of taking herbal remedies. Different parts of plants can be used to make tea. Gather a handful of whatever leaves, bark, stems, or roots that are needed, and boil them in one liter of water for about ten minutes. Drink the tea as needed. If the tea is for healing, as soon as the symptoms go away, you must stop drinking the tea.

Tincture

Tinctures are made with alcohol to preserve the herbs. If the tincture is to be applied to the skin, it is made with rubbing alcohol. If it is made to drink, it is soaked in white rum. Collect the parts of the herbs that you will use. Chop the herbs and soak in the alcohol for a week, shaking daily. Use in small amounts like a teaspoon every four hours. To drink the tincture, dilute a teaspoon in a glass of water.

Tonic

Drink chaya juice. Blend three or four big chaya leaves and add half a liter of water. Strain or filter and drink it. Add sugar or honey if desired, or drink it straight. Drink three or four glasses for the day. Boil cohune roots for a blood tonic. Boil a handful in one liter of water for about ten minutes. Drink four glasses for the day. Sorosi can also be used for a tonic to clean the blood for the immune system. Boil a handful of sorosi vine (stem and leaf together) and drink one glass every day.

Remedies for Common Illnesses and Complaints

The following are specific remedies that I use for the most common complaints of my patients. If a patient has been sick for a long time, I ask how long and treat the patient for one quarter of that time.

AIDS

Boost the immune system using the following recipes each day.

1) Make tea with contribo stem and palo de hombre leaves. Drink one glass daily.

2) Combine one leaf each papaya, cecropia, and piss-a-bed. Add eight leaves of polly redhead, and half a noni leaf. Boil in one liter of water and drink one glass per day.

3) Blend one ripe noni in half a liter of water. Add two teaspoons of milk and honey or sweetener to sweeten. Add ice to cool and drink the half liter through the day.

4) Drink one glass of chaya juice daily.

Allergies

Pelatum piper is used to treat allergies. Soak one mashed leaf in a glass of water for half an hour and then drink it. For severe allergies, drink two glasses for the day; for mild allergies, drink one glass for the day. If there are rashes from the allergies, bathe in mashed hog plum leaves. The hog plum bark can be boiled and drunk as a tea.

Anemia

Tea made with palo de hombre leaves or stems, sorosi leaves, cohune root is used to treat anemia because it strengthens the blood. Chaya juice also strengthens the blood.

19

Anger

A bath made from cockspur leaves is used to relieve anger. These trees have ants living in the thorns. Collect three of the ants on a Friday and let them bite the veins in the crook of the arm. Those ants are sucking out all your anger. Repeat with the other arm, and repeat with both arms two more times.

Arthritis and Rheumatism

We believe that arthritis (*can'il*) is caused with sudden changes of hot and cold. If you remove your shoe so your foot is hot and walk on the cold floor; if you bathe with a warm shower and then pour cold water on yourself; or if your hands are in cold water and then you put them in hot water: any of these can cause arthritis. Too much exposure to cold like washing laundry in the cold river water for hours at a time can cause arthritis.

Apply an ointment (*bok*) or tincture of the following leaves: yaxle'e, angel's trumpet, avocado, kach okpitch, ko'mo' che', at least two pipers, and wild grape to the joint two or three times a day. Use at least two if all of them are not available. This herbal ointment is excellent for strain, pain, arthritis, rheumatism, inflammation, mild stroke, and paralysis.

Asthma

We believe that asthma begins as a cough that is not taken care of, so the body accepts the cough as a part of it. Getting wet with cold water when you have a cold or cough can prolong it in your body and end up with asthma. There are several treatments for asthma:

1) Apply the arthritis ointment to the chest, throat, upper back, and on the wrists, especially at night.
2) Rub the chest with oil made from frijolillo leaves.
3) Drink one tablespoon cough syrup (*p. 12*) every four hours through the day for at least six months. If severe, drink through the night.

Athlete's Foot

We believe that exposure to polluted water, and too much closed up shoes or boots so the toes are wet and not exposed to fresh air, can both cause athlete's foot (fungus).

To clean and smooth fungus-infected toes and nails, use an ointment or tincture of alambre, cedar bark, yemeri bark, polly redhead, philodendron, ko'mo' che', and jackass bitters. Wash and dry infected toes and nails thoroughly, and then rub ointment or tincture on the area both morning and evening.

Bad Spirits and Bad Luck
Rudah is a good luck plant. It is used in baths, or soak the mashed leaves for half an hour, filter, and drink the water. This drink can also be used to sprinkle around to bless a business.

Balance
When off balance, either bathe with worm bush leaves or make a tea from the leaves and drink it.

Beef Worm
Copal can be used to suffocate the beef worm (bot fly larva) living under the skin. Put copal over the breathing hole and the larva will die. The glue from the leaves of the glue tree can be used to extract the botfly larva. The glue is placed on a small piece of paper to cover the breathing hole. This cannot get wet before the larva dies or it will not hold. The glue can be put on tobacco instead of paper. Clear nail polish, Vicks, or any ointment that is thick enough can also be used to seal off the breathing hole.

Behaviour Problems
Friolillo branches can be used to pass over children who are stubborn or won't listen. The branch is then thrown in the river. Or they can bathe with the same leaves.

Bleeding
Tea made from avocado, hibiscus, alepa or any citrus leaves can heal bruises and internal hemorrhages. If your blood is too thin, these teas will reduce bleeding. Drinking the juice of one lime squeezed in one glass of water normalizes the blood thickness, whether too thick or too thin. The smell of copal resin heals hemorrhages of the nose. Mixed with salt, animal fat will heal bruises.

Blood Pressure

Tea from the leaves of the hamans or cecropia normalizes blood pressure. Drink two glasses per day to normalize blood pressure whether it is low or high. Collect papaya leaves early in the morning, smash the leaf until the liquid starts to come out of the leaf, collect the liquid in a tablespoon and drink it.

Blood Purifier

Whenever you see discolouration of the skin, you need a blood purifier. But it is good to take a blood purifier at least two times for the year to keep healthy. Use any of the following recipes in January and June. We do it in January because during the holidays we tend to eat more sweets than any other time of the year. And in June because it is the middle of the year.

1) Bucut—dry the leaves and drink it as a tea, at least two glasses per day for one week.

2) Ix cat (wild cucumber)—drink bark tea, one glass per day for one week.

3) Jackass bitters—drink leaf tea, one tablespoon three times a day for two weeks.

4) Sorosi—drink vine and leaf tea, one tablespoon three times a day for two weeks.

5) Contribo/Waco—drink vine tea, one glass per day for at least a week.

6) Palo de hombre—drink leaf or stem tea, two tablespoons per day for two weeks.

Breast Feeding

The water from boiling young shoots of basket tie-tie spread on a new mother's breast will help her produce more milk. The mother's breast can be washed with the water in which corn was cooked with limestone to help the milk flow. Massage the breast with a comb downwards to activate the muscles and help with the flow. Drink a lot of corn porridge and cacao drink to make the milk flow.

Burns

Soak the inner part of the aloe vera leaf in water for 30 minutes and apply to burned skin. Gumbolimbo bark or leaves can be boiled with sugar and applied to burns and poisonwood burns. For burns from poisonwood, mango resin, or pepper, use sugar water to heal.

Cancer

We believe cancer is a bad spell that someone else wishes on you, or that you are just bad lucky. We believe that you can avoid it by taking care of yourself, eating healthy food, respecting other people, treating others with love, giving thanks to the Creator every day, being conscious of what you are doing, and having a positive outlook on life.

For treatment of cancer, drink at least one of these teas every day, whatever is easiest to get.

1) Cancer herb (whole plant) — drink at least two glasses per day.

2) Jackass bitters (leaf) — take one tablespoon in the morning and evening.

3) Hog plum bark and soursop leaf — drink one glass daily.

4) Calawala root and sorosi vine and leaf — drink one glass per day.

5) Ceiba leaves and thorns ground into a poultice or an ointment — use to treat external tumors.

6) Cleanse the aura twice per week by holding your hands on top of your head about two inches from your skin. Use a deep concentration and deep breathing, think of nothing else, and move the hands slowly down in front of the face and pass them in front of the body, then each side, then all the way down to your feet. Then do the same thing down the back, whatever you can do. Finally pass the hand over the other arm and out the hand, and have a motion of throwing away. If inside, open a window so you can throw it out the window. Repeat with the other arm. Repeat the whole process at least three times. If you can do it nine times, it is better. It helps to burn incense while cleansing the aura.

Cold, Cough, and Flu

We believe that we catch cold or flu when we get exposed to hot and cold. When the mattress is warm and you get up and go outside where it is drizzling and get cold, you might get sick. Being around people who have cough and cold, you can catch it. Exposure to excessive cold due to air-conditioning, especially when you are asleep, can make you catch cold.

Whenever the first symptoms of cold appear in the throat, make a salad of six oranges, add a pinch of powdered hot peppers, or mashed hot peppers, any kind, add a little salt, mix and eat it all. Repeat every day if necessary. Usually one bowl of salad is enough to avoid the cold.

Drinking the juice of one lime in a cup of hot water each day will help to avoid the cold or treat it. It is also good for a hoarse throat. Avoid drinking anything with ice.

If you catch the cold or flu, follow at least one of these remedies:

1) Lemongrass, cotton, or cha'al che' leaf tea.

2) Ginger root tea — mash an inch of ginger root, boil in half a liter of water for about ten minutes. Strain, sweeten with honey and add milk, if desired, and drink the tea.

3) Ironwood bark tea has lots of vitamin C — use for cough, cold, and fever.

4) Arthritis ointment — for a bad cold or flu, apply to the chest, throat, upper back, and on wrists, especially at night.

5) Frijolillo leaf oil — rub the chest with the oil.

6) Rabbit's paw leaf ointment — rub the forehead with ointment for sinus problems or drink a tea made from the leaves.

7) Cough syrup (*p. 12*) — take one tablespoon every four hours through the day until the symptoms are gone. If severe, drink through the night.

8) Bird peppers — eat to disinfect the throat.

Contraception

Drink avocado tree bark or seed tea for seven days before the menstrual period as a contraceptive. Repeat every cycle to prevent pregnancy.

Drink red hibiscus tea for a week during ovulation, beginning about ten days after the menstrual period. Repeat every month.

Dehydration

Coconut water from green coconuts can be used to rehydrate a dehydrated person. A poultice of piper leaves with ground cacao and eggs wet with alcohol can be placed on the palm of the hand, the bottom of the foot, and the forehead. Bathe with the same piper leaves boiled and add cold water to make a warm bath. Chaya juice is good for rehydration. Teas made from callaloo, palo de hombre, sorosi leaves, or any green herb that is edible will help to rehydrate a dehydrated person.

Depression

We believe that depression comes from being possessed with evil spirits or that a spell has been cast upon you. We believe that they can use your animals like your chickens to cast a spell on the family, or they can send bad spells with animals and birds, or even a powder of them. It is said that there is a lizard they use. Or they can use clothes that have your sweat, such as, underwear. You can get contaminated from other persons who have it. So the remedy is to cleanse from the evil spirits in all of the following ways:

1) Bathe with leaves of madre cacao, rudah, basil, ix tuc'ulil, and pipers for a total of nine species.

2) Drink zorillo macho root and stem tea, one glass per day.

3) Drink ix cat bark tea, one glass daily.

4) Bathe in the river and get nine rocks. Sit facing the river coming to you and pass the nine rocks over your body and throw them one at a time back downstream of the river. You can do this also if you have sadness from losing a family member. This works for getting rid of anything negative.

5) Smudge yourself by burning copal with a pinch of sage, sugar or honey, cinnamon, tobacco, and garlic in the early morning.

Diabetes

We believe that diabetes is caused by too much worry. Diabetes is *tuculil* in Mopan Maya and *tucul* in Yucatc Maya, both meaning "to worry."

To avoid diabetes, take one tablespoon jackass bitters in the morning and evening for a week two times a year.

To treat diabetes, boil one leaf each papaya, cecropia, and piss-a-bed, eight leaves of polly redhead, and half a noni leaf in one liter of water and drink one glass per day.

Digestion Problems

To treat diarrhea, use one or more of the following:

1) Allspice seeds — crush about 8 seeds, boil them in a cup of water, and drink.

2) Cashew leaves or bark — drink tea.

3) Craboo, monkey apple, or guava bark — drink tea.

4) Bay cedar — boil the bark or wash the slimy material inside the bark and drink it.

We believe that indigestion comes because of stress and nervousness, when you are not at peace with yourself, or you don't eat on time. When eating a hot meal, it is not good to drink a cold drink afterward because that is how indigestion starts. These are remedies for occasional indigestion and for chronic indigestion.

1) Drink allspice tea (*naba kuuk*) three times a day.

2) Use six leaves of wild oregano because it is a strong tea. Boil for five minutes in one glass of water. Drink the whole glass early in the morning before breakfast each day for a whole week.

3) Make ginger root tea with one inch square. Mash and boil in half a liter. Drink it all in one day. Make it each day for a whole week.

4) Drink basil leaf tea, about seven leaves boiled in one glass of water early in the morning before breakfast.

5) Pineapple and papaya juices help with digestion.

If indigestion is chronic:

1) Use the palo de hombre and contribo together. Boil a handful of the two combined together in one liter of water and drink at least one glass per day for at least eight days.

2) For chronic indigestion, I recommend a massage of the digestive system. It is done early in the morning before breakfast when the stomach is empty and has a prayer that goes along with it.

For gastritis, indigestion caused by gas, drink tea made from wild oregano leaves before breakfast.

For bellyache, drink tea made from the leaves of small oregano before breakfast.

For dysentery and infections in the digestive system, tea made from negrito bark acts as a disinfectant.

Ears

Crush culantro, thick oregano, and polly redhead leaves, cook in cohune oil, strain, and use one or two drops in the ear every day for ear infection.

Cecropia stem can be heated with fire to extract the juice, which is put in the ear to cure deafness.

Evil Eye

Babies can be hurt by a person watching the baby without holding them, or if they like a baby too much and don't hold the baby. The evil eye, or *malo de ojo,* can make the baby sick without the person being conscious of what is happening. Holistic baths with mallard stone or basil are used to treat the evil eye.

Eyes

To cleanse the eyes, we put about four basil seeds in the eye before going to sleep. In the morning all the dirt will come out along with the seeds. Or, scrape your own fingernail into a fine dust, drop it into the eye, and that will cleanse the eye.

For cataracts and other eye problems, we add a drop of honey from non-stinging bees, *doncella.*

If the sap of the poisonwood tree gets into eyes, the juice of the staircase plant leaves freshly mashed in water gives rapid relief.

Fever

We believe that fever is when you are tired and your immune system is getting low or weak. You can get fever when you are getting unbalanced spiritually, when somebody frightens you and you jump.

For fever, smash the leaf of the castor oil plant leaf (*ko'och*) and sprinkle the alcohol or rum on the leaf and wrap it around the palms of both hands, bottom of both feet, and around the top of the head. It sucks the fever out of the body and doesn't allow it to go into the head. Leave it overnight. The castor oil plant is very poisonous, so it must not be taken internally.

Frijolillo can be used as a bath. Boil two handfuls of frijolillo leaves in two liters of water for ten minutes and add cool water until it is warm for bathing. Pour it over the whole body, and leave it to dry, but don't rinse.

Drink palo de hombre tea made from either the leaf or the vine, but not both. For children, give one tablespoon every four hours. For adults, give one glass once a day.

Drink as much lemongrass tea as possible, both children and adults. Add sugar or honey and milk, if desired.

Allspice leaf tea normalizes body temperature, so it is good for fever.

When the fever becomes chronic, smudging helps, but you have to add a piece of your hair to the burning copal.

General Health

Drink tamarin or noni juice to maintain general good health. Ginger root mashed and made into tea is good for overall health. Add aloe vera leaf gel to food and eat it. Drink tea from either the leaves or stem, but not both, from palo de hombre because it strengthens the blood against diseases, especially diabetes and malaria. Tea made from young mango leaves are used to prevent coughs. Bathe with hog plum leaves for general hygienic cleansing. Mutazai philodendron is used as a bath for nine-month old babies to strengthen their bones so they walk sooner. But do not take mutazai internally because it is poisonous.

Hair

For hair conditioner, soak crushed leaves in water for half an hour. Use at least three of these leaves, whatever is available: young cacao, hibiscus, pita haya, prickly pear, malva, calawala, and cola de mico. After you finish washing your hair, wet the hair with the conditioner and leave it to dry without rinsing.

For a hair regrowth tonic (*tzak pol*) grind the same leaves as above together. Cook a handful in a liter of oil with a very low fire for a half an hour. Strain it. Apply every day before you comb your hair.

For dry hair, mash an over-ripe avocado and put it in your hair before you wash it. Leave it for ten minutes, then wash your hair. It makes the hair silky without tangles. Cohune oil can be used to maintain the colour of the hair.

Headache and Migraine

We believe that headaches come from too much worry and stress. Sleeping with wet hair can cause migraine headache or sinus problems. Wind can cause a headache if it hits your head.

There are several ways of treating headaches:

1) Castor oil plant—mash one leaf and sprinkle it with alcohol. Put it on your head and tie it. Do not take internally because this plant is poisonous.

2) Prickly pear leaf—split the leaf into half and tie it on the forehead.

3) Any of the small-leaf pipers (not big leaves like cowfoot) and verbena—soak either together or one at a time in water for half an hour. Tilt your head back and pour the water back over your head. Make a tincture and rub your head backwards with it three times per day.

4) The smell of copal resin removes headaches.

5) Smudge as described on page 17.

6) Release the tension by acupuncture. First have the person get some exercise to get the blood flowing. Then pierce the scalp in several places, four on the forehead in a cross shape and three more on the sides of the head. Put a towel over the head and apply pressure.

Hepatitis

Tea made from the bark or root of the wild cotton tree or piss-a-bed leaf or root is used to treat hepatitis (yellow jaundice), or bathe with piss-a-bed or monkey apple leaf. Hepatitis is also treated by eating the monkey apple fruit.

Immune System

To boost the immune system, scrape the inner part of aloe leaves, mix with food and eat every day.

Infertility

Cowfoot leaf tea is used to treat fertility problems. Drink palo de hombre leaf or contribo vine tea during the menstrual flow to increase fertility. Repeat at least three cycles.

Inflammation

Local inflammation that might come from an injury, like a sprained ankle, can be treated with herbal ointment made with at least two pipers, yax le'e, and ko'mo' che' or wash the affected area with cooled tea from the same leaves. Freshly mashed thick oregano leaves can be put on any inflamed area. A tincture or ointment made from siempreviva leaves is used to treat inflammation. Drink cowfoot tea or wet the area to treat inflammation.

For foot swelling from poor circulation or kidney problems, use the same ointment made from pipers, yax le'e, and ko'mo' che'. Make polly redhead, piss-a-bed, and cecropia leaf tea, the three combined, and drink at least two glasses per day.

Laxative

Castor oil plant seeds are ground to extract the oil to make a natural laxative. Drink a few tablespoons followed by a glass of milk early in the morning to flush out the system. After two or three hours when the system is sufficiently clean, eat some biscuits or tortillas to stop the flushing. After another three hours, eat a vegetarian or chicken soup to re-hydrate yourself. While using this technique, only shower in warm water and avoid the rain to avoid inflammation of the body.

Eat papaya fruit to improve digestion. Grind papaya seeds, boil them five minutes in water, filter, and drink one tablespoon in one glass of water as a laxative. To make more of a laxative, add oil, especially castor oil.

Menopause Hot Flashes

Allspice leaf (*naba kuuk*) tea balances the hormones, so it is good for menopause.

Menstruation

Contribo/Waco stem tea can be used to normalize menstrual flow. Hierba buena leaf tea decreases menstrual flow. Tea from cha'al che' leaves is used to treat menstrual cramps. Tea made from guava leaves is used as a douche.

Mumps

A tincture or ointment made from siempreviva or thick oregano leaves is used to treat mumps by putting it directly on the swelling.

Muscle Weakness and Paralysis

We believe that paralysis is caused by negative energies brought by wind, and heat and cold.

Bathe with leaves of ko'mo' che', rudah, basil, ix tuc'ulil, and pipers for a total of nine species, as hot as you can stand it.

Muscle Cramps

Bathe with tiger fern leaves.

Pain

Herbal ointment made with at least two pipers, whatever is around your area, and ko'mo' che' can be applied topically where the pain is.

A tincture or ointment of yaxle'e is used for pain.

Drink either palo de hombre, jackass bitters, cowfoot, or sorosi tea, one glass every four hours until the pain is gone.

Pregnancy and Delivery

Drink juice made from chaya leaves when pregnant. Coconut water and policacia leaf tea are good for women who have premature contractions to help hold the baby in place.

Just after birth, women are washed with tea made with guava leaves to clean them faster, dry quicker, prevent infection, reduce inflammation, and release pain.

Drink one cup of tea made from cha'al che' every day for a week after giving birth. For birth pain, drink policacia tea, one glass every four hours until the pain is gone.

Hog plum leaf tea is used for pain and infection, fibroma, or cysts in the womb.

Protection

Three pairs of cockspur thorns are tied with a red ribbon or cloth in a criss-cross pattern to hold them together. This is hung in front of the door of the house for protection from evil spirits or anything else negative. Give-and-take palm is used to sweep the house and that removes everything negative.

Purge

The oil made from castor oil plant seeds can be used as a purge once a year. But it has to be done during the dry season because the purge is hot and if you wet yourself after a purge, it can cause inflammation of the body. Tea from chicle bark also cleanses the blood and digestion.

Skin Lesions

For leishmaniasis (*chiclera*), make a tincture with jackass bitters, ko'mo' che' leaves, yemeri bark, hierba preniada, cha'al che', yaxnik, philodendron, and bucut. Wet a cloth with it and put it on the affected area. This remedy also works for ringworm, scabies, skin cancers, sores that won't heal, bed sores, grangrene or hair lice.

The resin from the red incense tree is put directly on leishmaniasis lesions. The slimy substance inside bay cedar bark can be washed off and used fresh to apply as a poulstice on leishmaniasis lesions.

For ringworm infections or tarantula bites, roast limestone and squeeze lime juice onto the hot powdered limestone and apply it as hot as you can stand.

To treat poisonwood rash, use tea made from gumbolimbo (bark or leaves), zorillo macho, jackass bitters, and staircase plant. If poison-wood gets in the eyes, use sugar water (one tablespoon of sugar in half a glass of water).

For prickly heat rashes and any other skin rashes or insect bites, make a tincture of jackass bitters, pipers, gumbolimbo, polly red-head, guava, bird pepper, lime, and any plum leaves. Apply on infected area twice daily. For external use only.

For heat rash, crush or grind young corn kernels, squeeze the juice, and put it to dry. Use the powder for heat rash.

For any skin rash put lime juice in bath water or treat with tea made with may plum leaves and bark.

For the red rash on newborn babies, put bird pepper leaf tea in the bath water.

For both a repellent and an anti-itch treatment for mosquito and other insect bites, make a tincture from beneno xut, jackass bitters, gumbolimbo, a few pipers, and polly redhead.

For scabes, make a tea from either zorillo macho, jackass bitters, or lime leaves. Apply on the area and drink it, too.

Treat warts with mango resin or red incense resin.

For dry skin, rub on cohune oil.

To make scars go away, make an ointment or oil from moses-in-the-cradle leaves.

Sleep Problems

Drink sensitive plant as a tea, three leaves in one cup of water, boil for five minutes, strain it and drink before you go to bed. Or bathe with it. We don't bathe babies with sensitive plant to help them sleep because it is said that the person will grow up to be lazy. Instead, we put a sensitive plant branch with leaves under the sheet. For adults, the branch would be under the pillow.

For babies who are not sleeping at night, bathe them with madre cacao.

A holistic bath is used to help with sleep issues. Allspice and zorillo macho tea also help with sleep problems.

Hierba buena is put it under the pillow or the sheet to stop nightmares.

Sore Throat and Tonsillitis

Gargle with a tea made with cotton leaves for a sore throat or tonsillitis.

Cough Syrup (*p. 12*) can also be used for a sore throat.

Boil onions and garlic, and gargle with the water for a sore throat.

Snakebite

The root of any piper can be used for snakebites. Mother-in-law tongue leaves are used as a poultice to treat snake bites.

Sprains

Pineapple leaves can be made into a tincture or an ointment to reduce swelling in sprains. Cowfoot leaf heated is tied with a piece of cloth on sprains.

Stomach Ulcers

Gumbolimbo bark tea sweetened with honey is used to treat stomach ulcers. Mallard stone leaf tea is used for stomach ulcers.

Stress

Make tea from ix tuc'ulil leaves, sour orange root, or the root of zorillo macho. Drink one cup per day. Or you can cut the leaves small, soak them for half an hour, and drink it fresh.

Ma'mu'kal leaves can be ground and put in oil to be spread on the skin as an energy booster, or ma'mu'kal can be used in a bath.

Bathe with one handful each of any piper and zorillo macho crushed and soaked in a bucket of water for three hours. Pour it from your head down until the bucketful is finished. Do not rinse. Use the pieces of the herbs to scrub your body. Any pieces that remain will drop off when your body dries.

Stroke (mild)

We believe that strokes are caused by wind, heat and cold, and stress. Sweep with a wild berry branch and then throw the branch away.

Massage with herbal ointment made with at least two of the pipers, whatever is available and ko'mo' che' mornings and evenings. Bathe as above for stress. Smudging helps with strokes, too.

Thorn

Copal can be used to help extract a thorn. Put a little bit of copal with the thorn and it will come out easily.

Tobacco Smoking Addiction

Cecropia leaves can be used to make Mayan cigarettes. Roll the leaves and set them in the sun for a few days to dry. They can be used to help remove a tobacco smoking addiction.

Toothache

For a toothache, gargle with a tea from pito or cowfoot leaves. Chewing piper leaves is very good for your gums. To extract a bad tooth, put a piece of copal inside the hole in the tooth and leave it. It will kill the root of the tooth and break it so it is easy to extract.

Trauma

Smudge and give prayer through the pulses. Bathe like for stress. Drink teas for the nervous system like allspice and zorillo macho. *Ensalmo (patz)* prayer is used to relieve trauma.

Tumor (non-malignant)

Grind the thorns and leaves from ceiba, boil them, and wash the tumor with the water. Or leave masa to get sour and add a little of the fat of the pig and salt. Spread on the tumor, which will make the tumor burst and then it can be cleaned so it will heal.

Urinary Problems

Teas from gumbolimbo bark, cancer herb, piss-a-bed, cecropia, and basil leaves are used to normalize urine flow and help the bladder. Any one of those, especially piss-a-bed, can be used for bed-wetting. Culantro leaf tea is a good diuretic.

Polly redhead leaf tea is used to treat bladder infections. Verbena leaf is dried first and then made into a tea to treat bladder infection.

Boil the roots of nine malva plants, a handful of mallard stone branches, and gumbolimbo bark together, and drink one cup a day for three days to produce excess urine to flush out kidney stones. Tea made from mosote stem or corn silk can be used to flush out kidney stones.

Corn silk boiled in water is used for other urinary problems. Make sure to hydrate yourself afterwards by drinking a lot of fluids.

Vision

Angel's trumpet flowers are hung in a bedroom if you want to dream to know your future. Put three Jesus Christ ferns, roots and all, in a glass of water, and put it under your bed to receive visions, if you want to know something that is unknown.

Weight Reduction

Hamans leaf tea helps to reduce the belly. Drink three glasses per day.

Eat only grapefruit for breakfast. Drink culantro tea early in the morning before breakfast to reduce appetite.

Worms

Jackass bitters tea works as a de-wormer or to purify your blood. Drink one tablespoon two times a day or twice a year just to improve your health and energize you. Palo de hombre, apasote, basil, contribo, small oregano, and zorillo macho leaves, and ginger root—any one of these made as a tea can be used as a de-wormer when drunk before breakfast. The soft tip on top of the stem and the leaves of cowfoot are used as a de-wormer.

Collect six leaves of soursop and boil in two cups of water and drink it before breakfast.

Prayers for balancing are part of the healing from worms. The condition of worms out of control in Mopan Maya is called *"hakil olal."* And in Yucatan Maya is *"hagan u yool."* Both mean that you are unbalanced.

Wound Healing

Chew acaliptus leaves and put it on a cut to stop the bleeding and hold it together like a stitch. When the wound heals, it will drop off.

Limestone powder on a wound will stop the bleeding. The dust on the new give-and-take palms can be scraped off and put on a wound to stop the bleeding, to seal it like a stitch.

Castor oil plant seeds are ground to extract the oil, which can be applied on top of a wound to facilitate healing. Cohune oil can also be used for wound healing. Polly redhead leaves can be roasted to soften them and the juice squeezed directly on a wound. Palo de hombre leaves can be pulverized to treat cuts and sores.

Tea made from bucut, cashew, golden plum, may plum, polly redhead, small oregano, thick oregano, guava, and hog plum leaves can be used as a disinfectant in wounds.

Craboo or chicle bark tea or tincture can help dry cuts or wounds.

Any animal fat, like pork fat or chicken fat, heals wounds quickly.

Herbal Plant Identification

This section contains descriptions and photos of the plants, their scientific names and their common names as we (author and editors) know them in English, Creole, Spanish, Mopan Maya, and Yucatec Maya. We have selected one common name for each plant to use thoughout the book. Others are listed in the descriptions of the plants. All the scientific and common names are listed in the index at the end of the book.

Scientific names are all in *Italics* and are composed of the *Genus* name and the *species* name, followed by the botanical author. The *FAMILY* name is in all capital letters on the upper right of each plant description. The medicinal plant descriptions and their uses are in alphabetical order by *Genus*.

In the descriptions of plants, one distinguishing feature is the configuration of leaves on a stem. Opposite leaves are directly across from each other. Alternate leaves on one side are between two leaves on the other side of the stem.

Leaves are often divided, sometimes more than once. The whole stem is a compound leaf and the small ones are called "leaflets." A coconut is a good example. The five-meter long stem is the leaf and the individual smaller ones are "leaflets."

In Mayan tradition, some species of plants are considered male and female counterparts, but they usually have the same medicinal uses. Those relationships are noted in the plant descriptions.

The editors were unable to scientifically identify 15 of the species, so they are listed alphabetically by the common name used in this book in the "Scientifically Unidentified Plants" section at the end of this chapter.

Below is an alphabetical list of the plant common names used in this book giving their *Genus* and *species* names and page numbers.

38

Common Name	Scientific Name	Page
acaliptus	unknown	140
alambre	*Lygodium venustum*	91
alepa	*Ipomoea sp*	82
allspice	*Pimenta dioica*	104
aloe	*Aloe vera*	45
angel's trumpet	*Brugmansia suaveolens*	53
apasote	*Dysphania ambrosioides*	73
avocado	*Persea americana*	100
basil	*Ocimum basilicum*	98
basket tie-tie	*Desmoncus orthacanthos*	70
bay cedar	*Guazuma ulmifolia*	79
beneno xut	unknown	141
bird pepper	*Capsicum frutescens*	56
bob	unknown	142
bucut	*Cassia grandis*	58
cacao	*Theobroma cacao*	134
calawala	*Phlebodium decumanum*	102
callaloo	*Amaranthus dubius*	46
cancer herb	*Acalypha arvensis*	43
cashew	*Anacardium occidentale*	47
castor oil plant	*Ricinus communis*	118
cecropia	*Cecropia peltata*	59
cedar	*Cedrela odorata*	60
ceiba	*Ceiba pentandra*	61
cha'al che'	*Pluchea carolinensis*	111
chaya	*Cnidoscolus chayamansa*	63
chicle	*Manilkara zapota*	93
cockspur	*Acacia cornigera*	42
coconut	*Cocos nucifera*	65
cohune palm	*Attalea cohune*	52
cola de mico	unknown	143
contribo	*Aristolochia trilobata*	51
copal	*Protium copal*	115
corazon	*unknown*	144
cordoncillo	*Piper jacquemontianum*	107
corn	*Zea mays*	138
cotton	*Gossypium hirsutum*	78
cowfoot	*Piper auritum*	106
craboo	*Byrsonima crassifolia*	55

culantro	*Eryngium foetidum*	74
frijolillo	*Senna occidentalis*	122
ginger	*Zingiber officinale*	139
give-and-take palm	*Cryosophila stauracantha*	67
glue tree	*Stemmadenia donnell-smithii*	131
golden plum	*Spondias mombin*	127
guava	*Psidium guajava*	116
gumbolimbo	*Bursera simaruba*	54
hamans	*Terminalia catappa*	132
hetero fern	*Lygodium heterodoxum*	90
hibiscus	*Hibiscus rosa-sinensis*	81
hierba buena	*Portulaca oleracea*	113
hog plum	*Spondias radlkoferi*	129
horse bush	unknown	145
ho'tz	unknown	145
ironwood	*Dialium guianense*	71
ix cat	unknown	146
ix tuc'ulil	unknown	147
jackass bitters	*Neurolaena lobata*	97
Jesus Christ fern	unknown	148
kach okpitch	*Adiantum concinnum*	44
ko'mo' che'	unknown	149
lemongrass	*Cymbopogon citratus*	69
lengua de vaca	unknown	150
lime	*Citrus aurantifolia*	62
madre cacao	*Gliricidia sepium*	77
mallard stone	*Phyllanthus amarus*	103
malva	*Sida acuta*	123
ma'mu'kal	*Porophyllum punctatum*	112
mango	*Mangifera indica*	92
may plum	*Spondias purpurea*	128
monkey apple	*Licania platypus*	87
moses-in-the-cradle	*Tradescantia spathacea*	135
mosote	*Priva lappulacea*	114
mother-in-law tongue	*Sansevieria hyacinthoides*	120
mutazai	*Philodendron hederaceum*	101
negrito	*Simarouba glauca*	124
noni	*Morinda citrifolia*	96
palo de hombre	*Quassia amara*	117
papaya	*Carica papaya*	57

pasmo	unknown	151
peltatum piper	*Piper peltatum*	105
pheasant tail	*Anthurium schlechtendalii*	50
philodendron	*Philodendron sp.*	101
pineapple	*Ananas comosus*	48
piper	*Piper* sp.	105, 108-110
piss-a-bed	*Senna alata*	121
pito	*Erythrina folkersii*	75
pita haya	unknown	151
policacia	unknown	152
polly redhead	*Hamelia patens*	80
prickly pear	*Opuntia cochenillifera*	99
rabbit's paw	*Sphagneticola trilobata*	125
red incense	*Tetragastris panamensis*	133
rudah	*Ruta chalepensis*	119
sensitive plant	*Mimosa pudica*	94
siempreviva	*Kalanchoe pinnata*	84
small oregano	*Lippia alba*	88
sorosi	*Momordica charantia*	95
soursop	*Annona muricata*	49
staircase plant	*Costus pulverulentu*	66
thick oregano	*Lippia graveolens*	89
tibush	unknown	152
tiger fern	*Dicranopteris pectinata*	72
tree fern	*Cyathea myosuroides*	68
verbena	*Stachytarpheta cayennensis*	130
wild berry	*Eugenia ibarrae*	76
wild cotton	*Cochlospermum vitifolium*	64
wild grape	*Lantana involucrata*	86
wild oregano	*Lantana camara*	85
worm bush	*Spigelia anthelmia*	126
yax le'e	unknown	153
yaxnik	*Vitex gaumeri*	136
yemeri	*Vochysia hondurensis*	137
zorillo macho	*Justicia breviflora*	83

Acacia cornigera (L.) Willd

cockspur, subin, bullhorn

Cockspur grows as a small tree in hilly areas such as the Toledo and Cayo Districts. Each leaf is divided twice with nine stems (25 cm), each with as many as 40 small (2 cm) opposite leaflets. Large (50 cm) thorns grow where the leaf comes off the main stem.

There are related species giving different fruits. This species has long beans that are black when ripe. Another species has oblong fruits (5 cm), that are reddish brown when ripe.

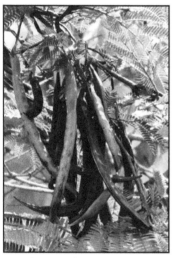 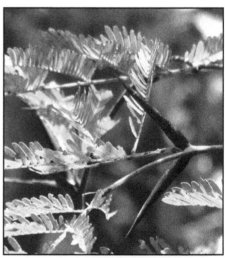

Both species are used in the same ways. The thorns are used in acupuncture. The leaves are used for holistic or sacred baths to bring in good energy. The ants that grow inside the tree are used as oil for the chest to cure asthma. The ants are used to treat depression by holding the ant in the crook of the elbow on a vein until the ant bites several times. The potent aroma from crushing the ants smells much like incense or copal oil.

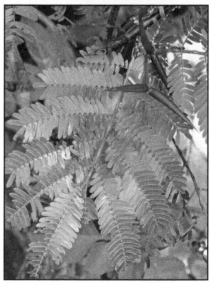

Acalypha arvensis Poepp.

cancer herb, hierba del cancer

Cancer herb has triangular leaves pointed at the tip and rounded at the base. The tiny pink flowers are on spikes sticking out of a ball. It grows mostly in open areas and flowers throughout the year.

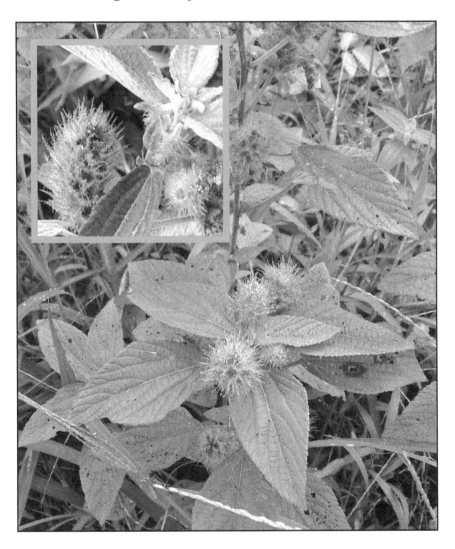

Tea made from cancer herb leaves is used to treat and prevent cancer, and for urinary problems. For skin cancer, wash with the tea.

Adiantum concinnum Humb. & Bonpl. ex Willd.

**kach okpitch, brittle maidenhair fern, polished maidenhair
fern**

Kach okpitch is a fern with up to 24 pairs of fan-shaped
leaflets with pointed bases and lobed outer edges. Because
the stem is dark, the light green leaves seem to float over
the ground. The leaves change colour beginning like the
yellowish green shown, then pinkish red and then green
when they are mature.

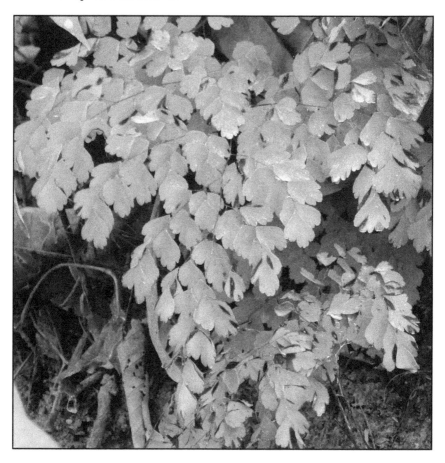

Kach okpitch is used in ointments to treat arthritis.

Aloe vera (L.) Burm. f.

aloe, sink-and-bible

Aloe is a succulent plant with long (20 cm), thick leaves with small spines on the edges. The leaves grow out of a base in a circular pattern, growing to 50 cm tall. Young leaves have small white spots. This plant does not grow in the wild in Belize. It is used for decoration as a good luck plant.

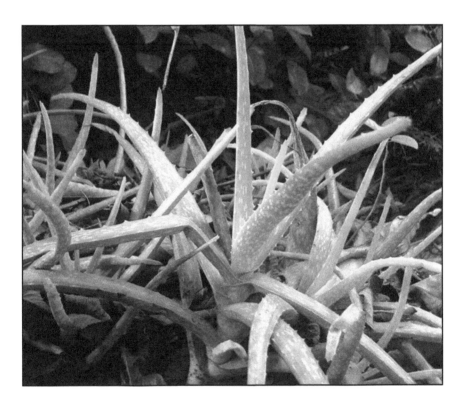

The gel inside aloe leaves can be spread on the skin to ease the pain of burns. The gel is eaten by mixing with food to protect health and to prevent pulmonary infections.

AMARANTHACEAE

Amaranthus dubius Mart ex Thell.

callaloo, calaloo, wild spinach, ix calalo

Callaloo is a shrub with many branches growing out of the center to one meter tall. The alternate leaves (10 cm long) are oval, round at the base with a pointed tip and smooth edges. The upper surface of the leaves is smooth while the lower surface is hairy. The green flowers are on branched spikes. Callaloo produces many black seeds.

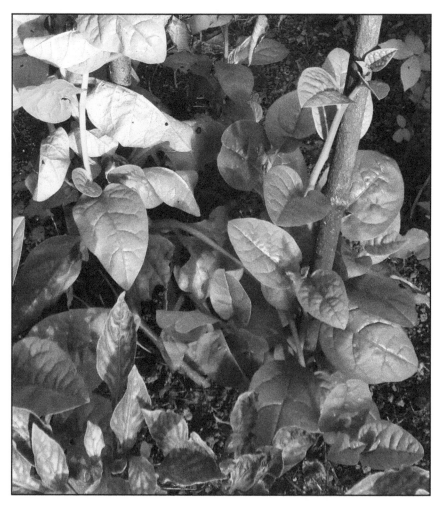

Tea made from callaloo leaves is used to treat dehydration.

Anacardium occidentale L.

cashew, maranion

Cashew grows as a tree as much as 15 meters tall with oblong leathery leaves with smooth edges and a rounded tip. The small pale green flowers grow in round clusters that turn reddish. The fruits are bright yellow with the seed on the outside. The seed must be roasted to destroy a potent toxin in the outer layer before it is edible.

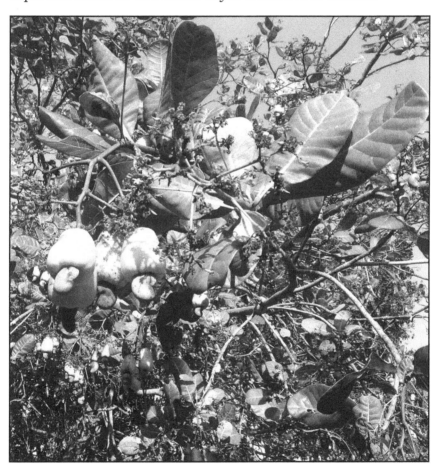

Tea made from cashew leaves or bark is used to treat diarrhea, or as a disinfectant in wounds.

Ananas comosus (L.) Merr.

pineapple, piña

Pineapple grows as a swirl of long (1.5 m) leaves originating at the ground level. The leaves are shaped like a trough with saw-toothed edges. The fruit grows from the middle of the swirl of leaves. The fruit is actually many fruits produced from individual flowers that join together. After the fruit is produced, side shoots called "suckers" that grow from the main stem can be used to grow new plants.

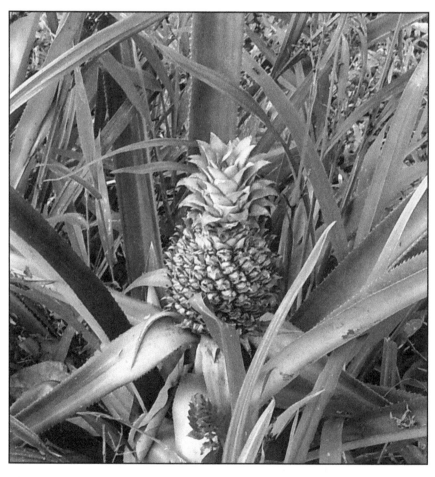

Pineapple juice is helpful for the digestive system. The leaves are used for tinctures and ointments, which are put on sprains to remove the swelling quickly, or to remove bruises.

Annona muricata L.

soursop, guanábana, wanabe'

Soursop grows as an evergreen tree with alternate shiny, oblong (25 cm) leaves with a pointed tip. The yellow-green flower that grows out of the stem or trunk is composed of three tough heart-shaped petals in each layer. The large green fruit is of variable shape with many thorns.

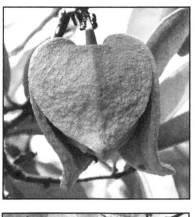 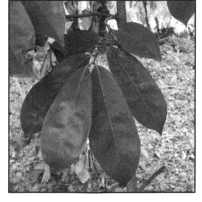

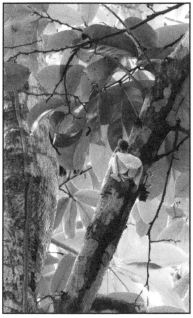 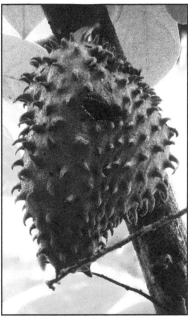

Tea made from soursop leaves is used to make cough syrup, to treat cancer, and as a de-wormer.

Anthurium crassinervium (Jacq.) Schott.

pheasant tail, corbata

Pheasant tail is an herb with large (1 m) oblong leaves with pointed tips and crinkly edges. The leaves grow from the ground all the way up. It is a wild plant commonly found around Mayan sites. The flower resembles a pheasant's tail.

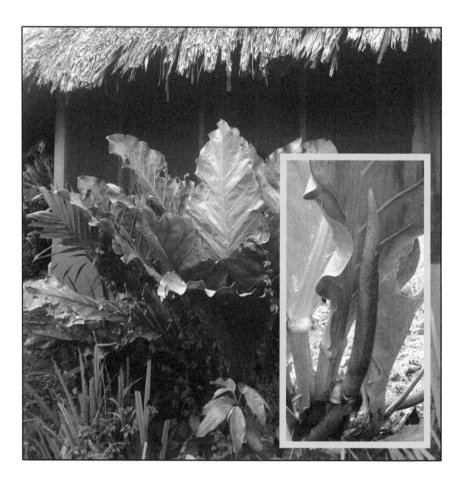

Pheasant tail is a sacred plant for the Maya that is used in enchanting and prayers, for spiritual and holistic baths, and for prayers on the pulse points of the body. The symbolism is to take away the negativity: sickness, nervousness, stress, whatever is the problem.

Aristolochia trilobata L.

contribo, duck flower, flor de pato, anjus a'ck

Contribo is a small vine with U-shaped leaves (20 cm long) that have a deep (5 cm) split at the base. The stem has straight rough strips on the back. The small flower of contribo is in the shape of a duck; it looks like an orchid, but is not an orchid. The contribo stem has a sweet scent like liquorice. This plant likes creek beds in the hilly regions like the Cayo and Toledo Districts.

The male counterpart to the female contribo is the waco, which has larger duck-like flowers that grow up to 15 cm long.

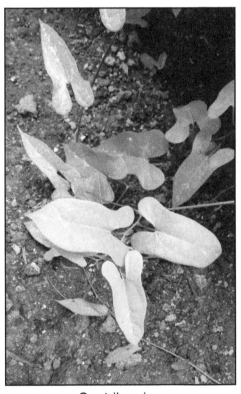 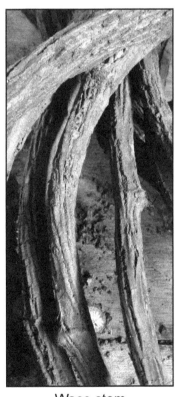

Contribo vine   Waco stem

Tea made from mature stems of contribo and waco is used as a blood purifier, for abdominal pains, stomach cramps, chronic indigestion, to normalize the menstruation flow, and to treat worm infections. It has also been used to treat infertility with great results.

Attalea cohune Mart.

cohune palm, tuz

This wild palm is one of the most useful plants in the Mayan culture. This is shown by the sheer number of them around Mayan temples. The palm leaves are very long (as much as 8 m). Cohune palms bear large bunches of nuts that can be eaten green off the tree or dry off the ground. The Maya break open the nut to reveal the kernel inside.

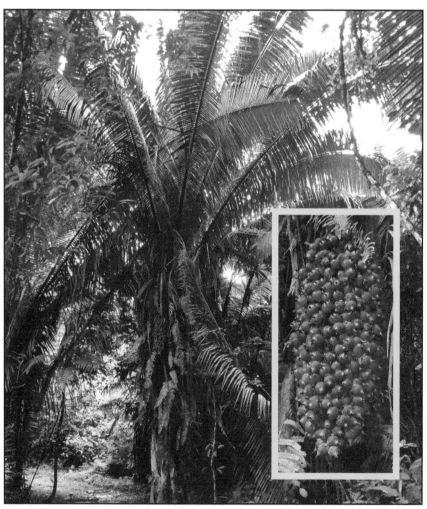

The oil can be used to make medicinal oils like those for hair, ears, or wounds. It is excellent for dry skin, treating hair, cooking, and for oil lamps. The roots of cohune palm are used for a tonic for blood.

SOLANACEAE

Brugmansia suaveolens (Humb. & Bonpl. Ex Willd.) Bercht
   & J. Presl.

angel's trumpet, datura, campana top'

Angel's trumpet is a tall woody shrub with large (25 cm
long) coarse, oval, alternate leaves that have either smooth
or toothed margins. The large (20 cm long) white and
trumpet-shaped flowers hang down. Flowers can also be
purple or pink.

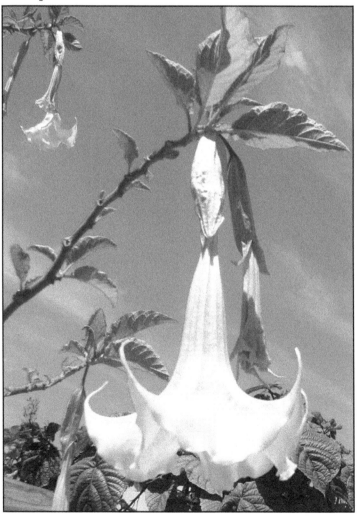

Angel's trumpet leaves are used in ointments for arthritis
and rheumatism. The flowers are hung in the bedroom to
induce prophetic dreams.

Bursera simaruba (L.) Sarg.

gumbolimbo, tourist tree, chaca'

Gumbolimbo is a tall tree with the trunk growing to as much as one meter in diameter. The compound leaves have three to seven opposite leaflets that are oblong with a pointed tip (7 cm long). The flowers are in a cluster at the top of the tree, so not often seen. The peeling red bark is unmistakable.

The red gumbolimbo is the female one. The white gumbolimbo is the male counterpart. It has the same way of flowering, except the peeling bark is white, not red.

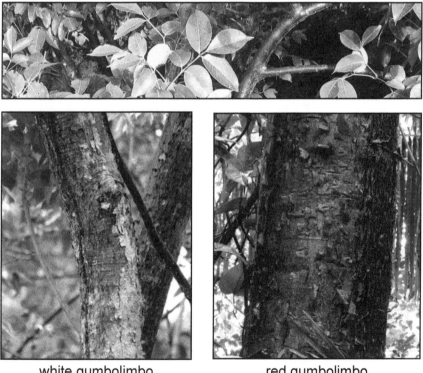

white gumbolimbo   red gumbolimbo

Gumbolimbo bark is used for tea to treat bladder infections, and flush out gall and kidney stones. Drink one cup a day. It is boiled and rubbed on infected areas four times a day to treat poisonwood rash, to ease the itch and stop spreading. Sweetened with honey, the gumbolimbo bark tea can be used to treat stomach ulcers. Drink one cup a day.

Byrsonima crassifolia (L.) H.B.K.

craboo, nance, chi'

Craboo is a tree that grows to seven meters with light-coloured rough bark. The oblong leaves (4-15 cm long) are clustered at ends of branches, glossy on the upper side and hairy on the underside with smooth edges. The small yellow and orange flowers with white centers are in clusters. Craboo produces the popular edible small yellow grape-like fruit (1.5 cm across).

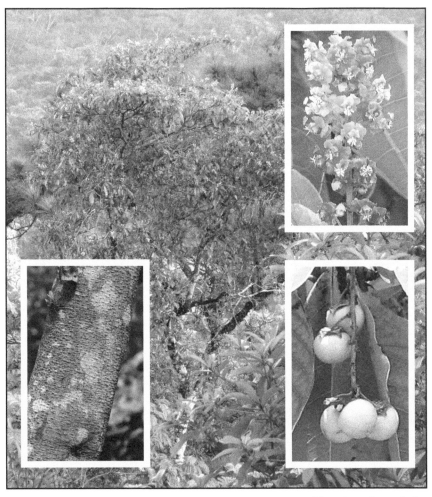

Tea made from the bark of craboo is very effective for plain diarrhea. Craboo bark or leaf tea or tincture is used for drying sores or cut wounds in the skin.

Capsicum frutescens L.

bird pepper, chili pepper, mash ik

Bird peppers grow as a bush with oval leaves (10 cm) pointed at the base and an elongated point at the tip and small pointed red or yellow fruit.

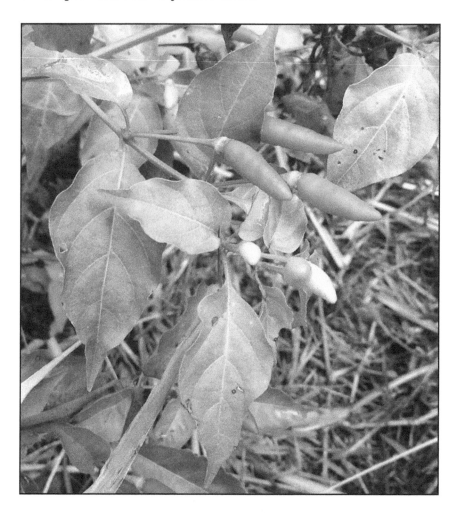

Tea made from the leaves of any bird pepper plant is used for skin rashes, such as heat rash, and especially the red rash on newborn babies. It can also be used to disinfect the throat.

These peppers are very hot, so you have to be very careful touching them, or you can burn your face or eyes.

Carica papaya L.

papaya, put'

Papaya has been domesticated to give large (40 cm) yellow fruit and grows throughout Belize. It grows as a small tree up to five meters tall. The large (50 cm) many-lobed, deeply toothed leaves are on long stems clustered at the top.

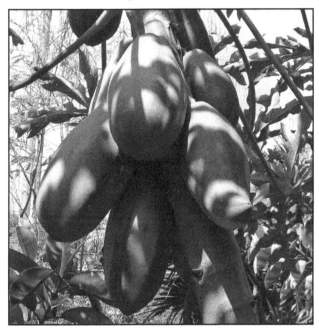

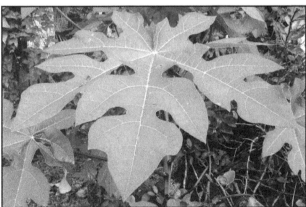

Papaya leaf tea is good for treating high blood pressure, diabetes, and AIDS. Its fruit and seeds can be used as a laxative. The fruit is helpful for quick digestion.

Cassia grandis L.

bucut, stinking toe

Bucut grows to a large tree with a long (50 cm) dark fruit and cascading light pink flowers, which come out before there are any leaves. The trees are often used as decorative trees in yards. The fruit is rich in iron and customarily made into juice. The compound leaf (40 cm long) is comprised of small, oblong leaflets (5 cm) with as many as 20 opposite pairs.

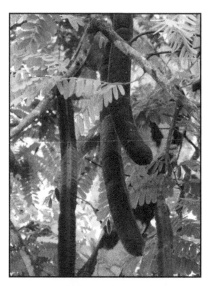

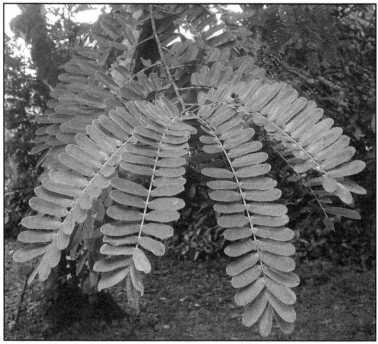

Tea made from bucut leaves is used to cure leishmaniasis (baysore or chiclera). Bucut leaves are also used for cleansing the blood and to treat sores. Tea made from bucut leaves dries wounds quickly and disinfects.

Cecropia peltata L.

cecropia, trumpet tree, warumo

Cecropia is a quick-growing tree, the first tree to grow in a newly opened space. It is recognized by the leaves with ten lobes and the light-coloured trunk with nodes.

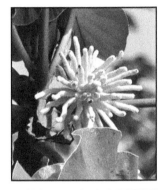

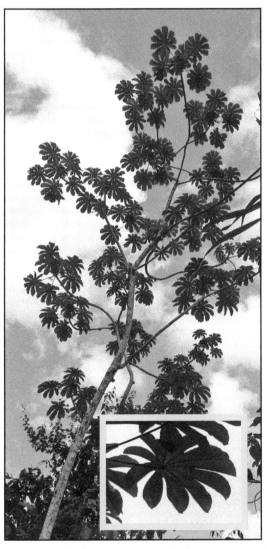

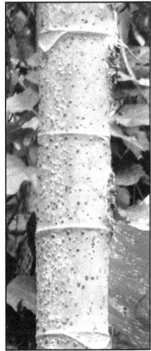

Tea made from cecropia leaves can be taken internally in small amounts to treat diabetes and inflammation. The cecropia stem can be heated with fire to extract the juice, which is put in the ear to cure deafness.

MELIACEAE

Cedrela odorata L.

cedar, cedro, ku' che

The cedar tree grows as tall as 30 meters. The trunk has grey bark, with irregular striations up and down. Each compound leaf is divided into approximately 20 opposite oblong leaflets that are pointed at both ends. The Mayan name means "the tree of the gods" because it is the wood that is used for carving statues of gods, so it is considered a holy tree.

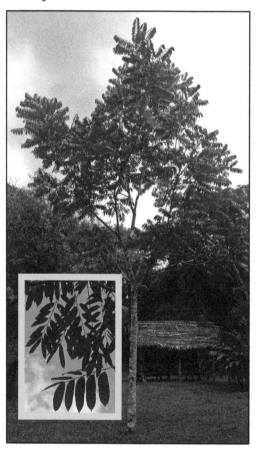 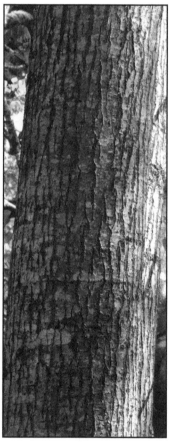

Cedar bark or leaves are used in ointments or tinctures to treat athlete's foot or other fungus infections. Tea from the bark can be drunk for asthma and pneumonia. When they are flowering, you can sit under the tree and smell the flower to stop nose hemorrhage. The aroma of the flowers is not nice, and it can be smelled from far.

Ceiba pentandra (L.) Gaertn.

ceiba tree, cotton tree, yax che'

Ceiba trees are among the largest in Belize. They are also called "cotton tree" for the cotton balls in which seeds are dispersed. The oblong leaves are pointed at both ends. The large trunks have buttress roots. The smooth trunk has cone-shaped thorns in clusters.

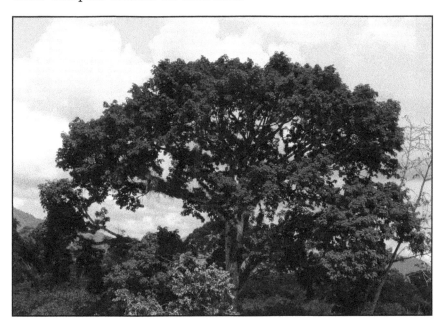

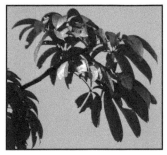
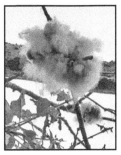
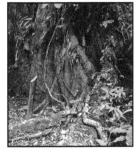

Ceiba trees are sacred to the Maya people. The ceiba tree is said to connect the three planes of sky, earth, and underworld. When a field is cleared, large ceiba trees are left.

Ceiba thorns and leaves are ground up and boiled to treat tumors, except the leaves are hard to get because the trees are so big. Ceiba thorns are used for acupuncture.

RUTACEAE

Citrus aurantifolia (Christm.) Swingle
lime, limon

Many varieties of lime trees exist in Belize. Most have thorns on the stems and leaves (5-15 cm) with pointed tips and smooth edges in an alternate configuration.

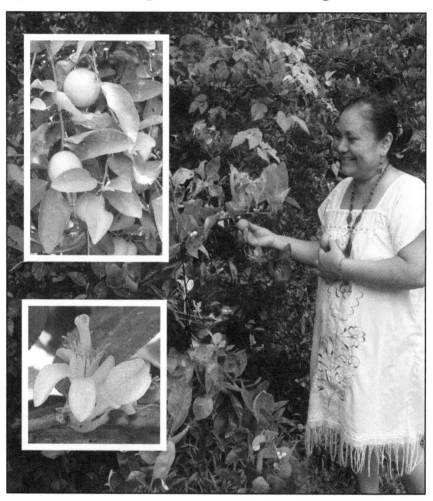

Because the they are full of vitamin C, fruits of lime trees are very good for coughs. You can put the juice in bath water to remove skin rashes. For tarantula bites and ring-worm infections, roast limestone, squeeze lime juice into the hot powdered limestone, and apply it as hot as you can. Lime is considered a cleansing plant, so whole fruits are hung at the entrance of businesses.

Cnidoscolus chayamansa McVaugh

chaya

Chaya is an evergreen climber with large round leaves with five to seven sharp points. It has small white flowers in a cluster at the top of a stem. *Cnidoscolus chayamansa* is the domesticated chaya that does not sting. *Cnidoscolus aconitifolius* is the wild chaya that has stinging hairs on the leaves, so if you see it in the wild, don't touch it.

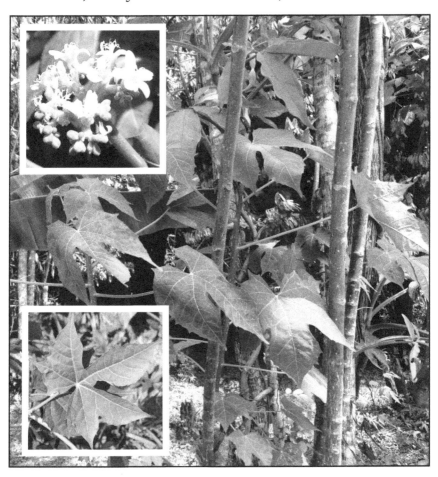

The leaves of this edible plant can be boiled or fried like spinach. The iron-rich juice made of the leaves is used as a tonic and especially recommended for pregnant women. The wild chaya is collected; the stinging hairs are scraped off; and the leaves are cooked slowly in oil. The oil is taken in small amounts for asthma.

Cochlospermum vitifolium (Willd.) Spreng.

wild cotton

Wild cotton grows to a medium tall tree with five-lobed oblong pointed leaves and saw-toothed edges, each vein ending in a small point. The bright yellow flowers develop into a spherical fruit with alternating light and dark brown sections. The fruit breaks open to release seeds embedded in cotton.

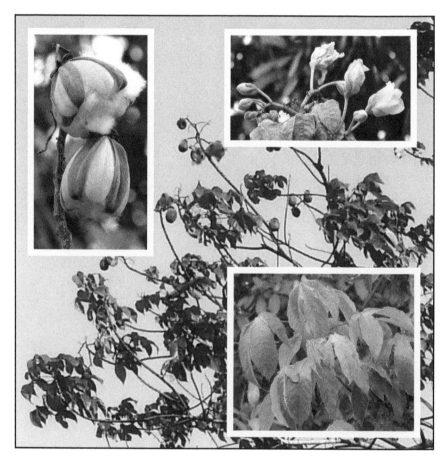

Tea made from wild cotton leaves are used to treat colds, flu, sore throats, hepatitis, and asthma, both by drinking the tea and bathing in it, including the flowers in the bath, if possible.

Cocos nucifera L.

coconut, coco

Coconut palms are found all over Belize. The leaves (6 m long) are divided into many long leaflets. The flowers come out in a large brown boat-like structure called a "shooty." The large green nuts form the basis of Belizean cuisine.

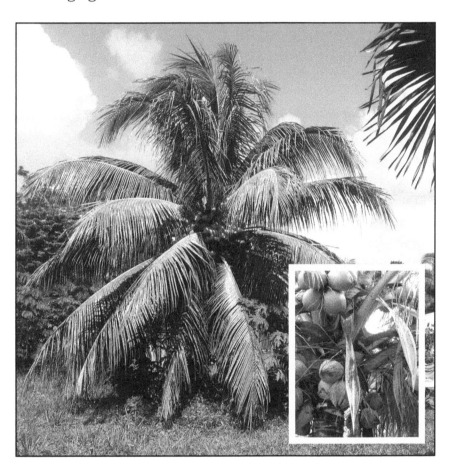

Coconut water in a green coconut is a refreshing juice that is great for dehydration or a high fever. When you are weak, drinking fresh coconut water will give you energy; it works like a drip. Coconut water can be made into medicine for women who have premature contractions to help hold the baby in place. The dried coconuts are used to make oils, which are very good for both skin and hair, and burn like kerosene.

Costus pulverulentus C. Presl.

staircase plant, costa plant

The staircase plant is very common in all of the tropical forests of Belize. The large leaves grow alternately off a single central stem as high as two meters, resembling a staircase. The waxy leaves (50 cm) have light stripes that parallel the edges and the central vein. The flower is a waxy red pointed knob (12 cm high) that grows out of the top of the stem. The plant grows along rivers and in open areas with plenty of sunlight. It is generally used as an ornamental and for gardening; however, its flowers can be used to make vegetable salad if enough are collected.

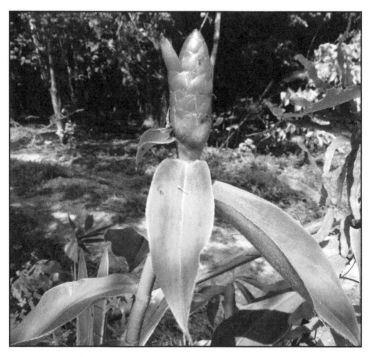

There are male and female plants which are separated only by the colours of the stems and the underside of the leaves. The male plants have red stems and the female has white stems. The female staircase plant is smaller and the male plant grows taller. Either can be used to heal the burning from the poisonwood (*chechem*) poison when the leaves are mashed in water and wet the infected area. Mayan children eat the stem of the plant as a source of vitamins.

Cryosophila stauracantha (Heynh.) R. Evans

give-and-take palm, broom palm, escoba, miis

Give-and-take palm grows to a tall tree with round fronds composed of many long, thin leaflets that work well as a broom. The stems have many long thorns. The heart of the palm is edible.

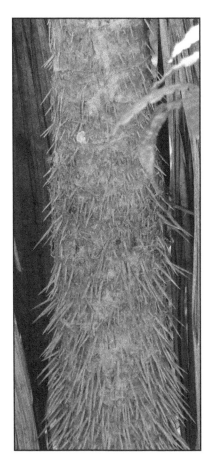
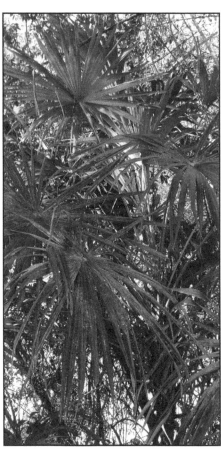

Give-and-take palm is used to stop bleeding. Scrape off the soft spongy brown dust that layers itself on the top center where the leaves come out and put it directly on the wound to stop bleeding.

Sweeping with the give-and-take palm gets rid of negativity. The thorns can be used for acupuncture.

Cyathea myosuroides (Liebm.) Domin
tree fern, helecho

Like other ferns, the tree fern stem and leaves unfurl from a structure called a "fiddlehead" for its resemblance to the end of a violin. The tree fern leaf is divided twice. The main stem (2-3 m) has 20-30 alternate stems (50 am), each with 20-30 small leaflets (1 cm) also in alternate configuration. When cut, the main stem has four cardinal points that serve as a compass for the Maya when in the jungle.

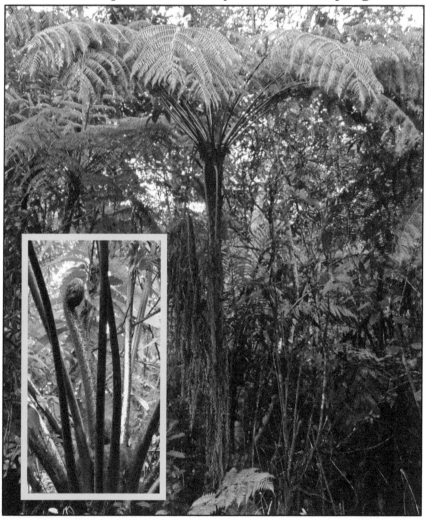

Tree fern leaves are boiled and used in warm baths to relieve elderly cramps.

Cymbopogon citratus (DC.) Stapf.

lemongrass, sacate' limon

Lemongrass is a grass that grows to about 50 cm tall in dense clumps. It is recognized by the lemon scent of the leaf.

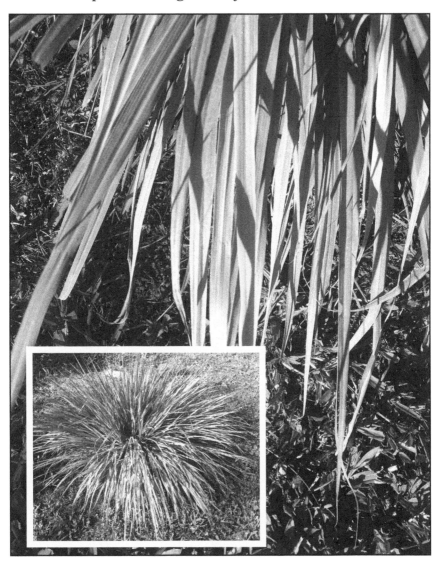

Lemongrass is rich in vitamin C, so lemongrass tea is used to treat cough, sore throat, fever, colds, and hay fever. Drinking lemongrass tea regularly is good to keep a person healthy.

Desmoncus orthacanthos Mart.

basket tie-tie, bayel, bayal

This very wicked looking plant is unusual for a number of reasons. Although it is a palm, it takes the form of a vine climbing upward over other forest trees. The entire vine is covered with small but sharp needle-like spines. The leaf tips are also modified into a series of reverse-hooked spines. By catching an animal's hair, the vine is passively moved across the forests and along pathways. Its name is derived from its principal use, basket-making.

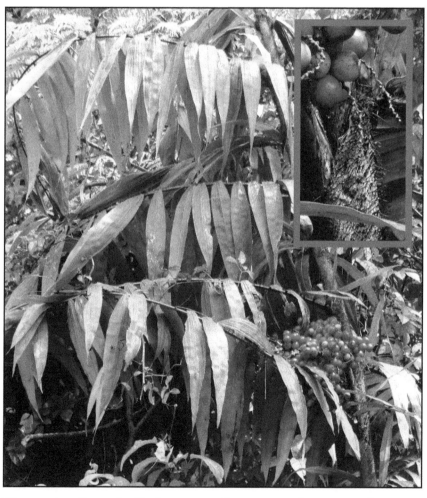

The water from boiled young shoots can be spread over a new mother's breasts to help her produce more milk.

Dialium guineense Willd.

ironwood, wild tamarin, chatchi, chate, palo de lacandon

A common tree in the Atlantic lowlands of Central America, ironwood gets its common name from its very hard, heavy wood. It may weigh up to 55 pounds per cubic foot and does not float. The compound leaves have alternate leaflets (3-7 cm long). It has low root buttresses from which it grows very straight. The green to brown fruits are marble-sized found in bunches.

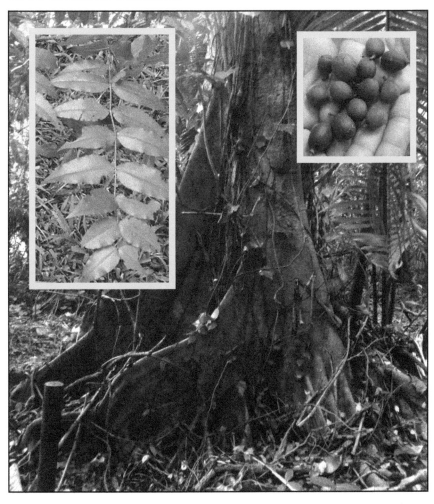

Maya children eat ironmoood fruit or drink its juice to maintain general health. Tea from ironwood bark has lots of vitamin C, so it is good for cough, cold, and fever.

Dicranopteris pectinata (Willd.) Underw.

tiger fern, culantrillo

Tiger fern grows in huge patches that can take over entire hilltops. As a fern, the divided leaves unfurl into a stem with 40 or more leaflets that are wider at the base and gradually decrease in width toward the tip.

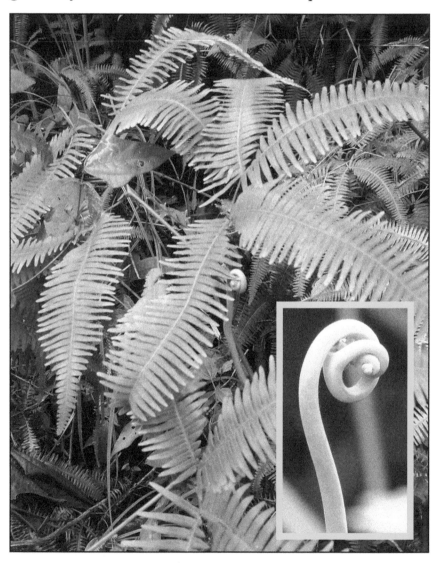

Tiger fern roots are boiled to be taken as a blood tonic for anemia because they are high in iron.

Dysphania ambrosioides (L.) Mosyakin & Clemants

apasote, epazote

Apasote is an aromatic kitchen herb growing to one meter tall with a hairy stem. The narrow leaves (10 cm) are rounded at the tip and pointed at the base. On the underside of the leaves are yellow glands. The very small greenish-white flowers grow on short spikes out of green nodes on the stems. The black seeds are less than 1 mm long and contain toxic oil.

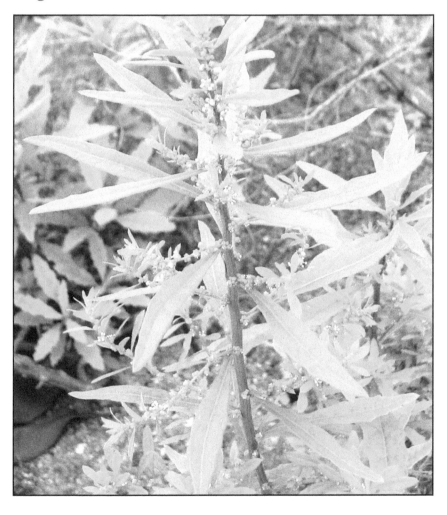

Apasote leaf tea is used as a de-wormer.

Eryngium foetidum L.

culantro, wild cilantro, cilantro simaron

Culantro leaves are oblong with rounded tips and serrated edges. The green flowers grow on central stems that have pointed, spikey petals with a central developing fruit. Culantro grows wild around yards in Belize.

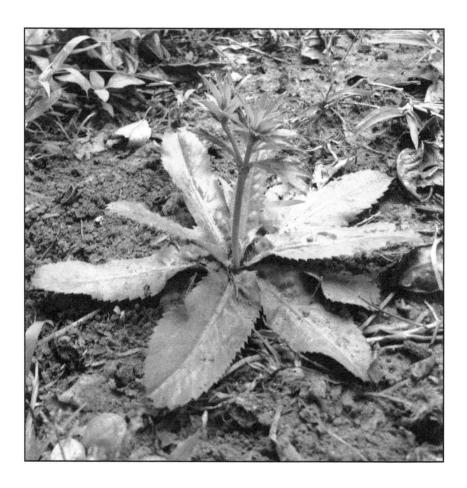

Culantro is used in salads and flavoring. When the leaves are boiled and drank like a tea, it is useful as a diuretic and for weight reduction. The leaves made into an oil are used for ear infections and earaches.

Erythrina folkersii Krukoff & Moldenke

pito, arbol de pito, pito coral tree

Pito grows as a tall bush with large triangular leaves with pointed tips and wide rounded bases at the ends of branches. A green bean is produced with six to nine seeds that turns dark as it matures and opens to reveal red and yellow seeds. Children make whistles from the flower, which accounts for the name "pito" that means "whistle" in Spanish.

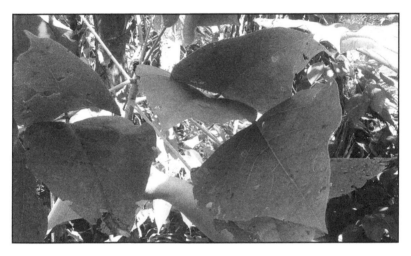

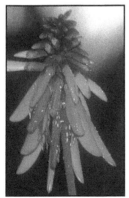
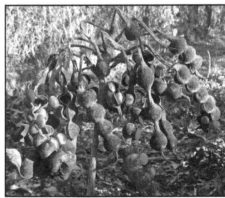

Gargling with tea made from the pito leaves is good for toothaches. The pito flower is edible. It is popular with the Maya when fried with scrambled eggs. The leaves are also good to eat because they have a lot of iron.

Eugenia ibarrae Lundell
wild berry, chillon che'

Wild berry grows as a small tree with opposite, waxy leaves pointed at the tip and rounded at the base. The fruits are small red and yellow berries, each on a short stem.

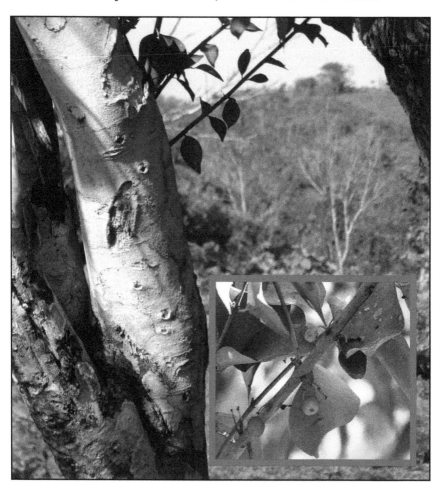

Wild berry is a sacred tree that is considered to have the power to remove negativity in a person. After a ceremony connecting with the gods, the priest uses a branch of wild berry to cleanse himself and the participants by brushing with it and then getting rid of the branch. Wild berry is used for mild strokes and paralysis the same way. The juice is drunk to treat measles.

Gliricidia sepium (Jacq.) Kunth ex Walp. or (Jacq.) Steud.

madre cacao

Madre cacao is a small tree (to 10 m) that is fast growing and will grow on sandy or rocky soils. It is used as a shade tree for cacao, which accounts for its name. The leaves are divided into stems with five to fifteen oval leaflets each. The light pink flowers hang down in clusters, usually on older branches after the leaves have fallen. There is another species that has a yellow flower that doesn't grow as big.

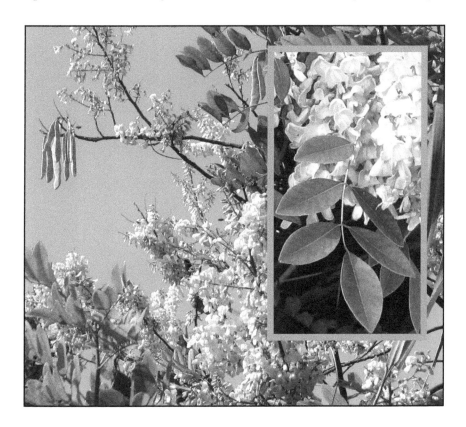

Madre cacao leaves are used for holistic baths and baths to purify, especially when babies are unable to sleep in the night.

Gossypium hirsutum L.

cotton, tumun, pitz

The domesticated cotton plant is also a medicinal herb that grows as a shrub. The alternate leaves (10 cm across) have three large points and sometimes one smaller point. Young leaves are round with a pointed tip. The rose-coloured flower is a tight rosy swirl. There are two species of cotton, one that has a lot of seeds throughout the cotton, and one that has seeds clumped in the center of the cotton.

Though this plant prefers dryer land, it can grow nearly everywhere in Belize and is very common in the northern districts.

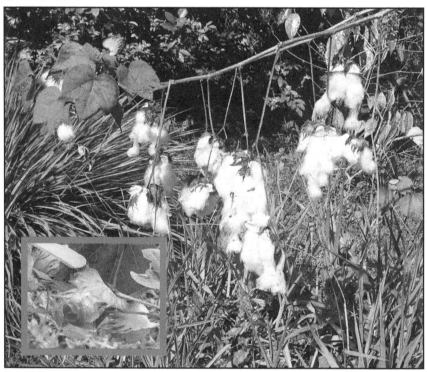

It is good to grow your own cotton to use in cupping because commercial cotton has other components and it will not light properly. Tea made from cotton leaves can be gargled to treat tonsillitis and inflammation of the throat. When the leaves are boiled and drank, it can prevent coughs for a year. The children like to suck on its young, sweet fruits.

Guazuma ulmifolia Lam.

bay cedar, tapaculo, pixoy

Bay cedars grow into big trees with alternate leaves that are finely serrated on the edges with pointed tips and rounded bases. The small white flowers are on branched stems that grow from the same nodes as the leaves. The fruits are black oblong spheres with many rounded spikes.

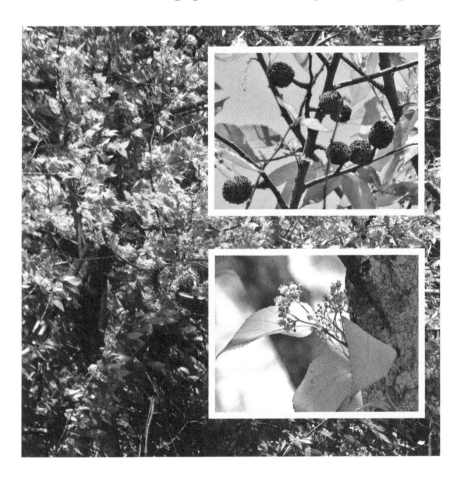

The fruits of the bay cedar tree are eaten when they are dry to stop diarrhea, which accounts for the Spanish name, "tapaculo." There is a slimy resin when you open the bark, so wash it into a glass to drink as a juice. This slimy resin is good for leishmanaisis. Or a tea can be made from the bark.

Hamelia patens Jacq.

polly redhead, red polywood, ix ka'nan

Polly redhead is an unmistakable shrub. The opposite leaves (20 cm) have a red vein in the center and red edges. The small red tubular flowers are in clusters on short stems throughout the year.

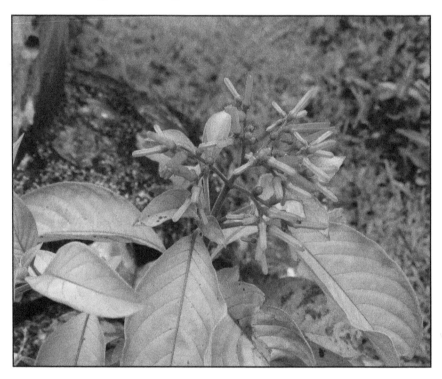

The leaves of this plant work as an antibiotic to heal sores, cuts and wounds. The leaves are boiled and the water used to wash the affected area. You may also roast the leaves on a grill to soften them and then squeeze the juice from the leaves directly onto the wound. Or, they can be made into a powder by drying leaves in the sun and then grinding them. Drinking the tea heals kidney infections or other infections anywhere in the body. Tea made from polly redhead mixed with cecropia leaves is good for diabetes. To build the immune system, soak polly redhead leaves and drink a glass of the water a day.

Hibiscus rosa-sinensis L.

hibiscus, tulipan

Hibiscus is popular as a decorative plant. These beautiful flowers are plentiful throughout Belize. The glossy, oval alternate leaves have serrated edges. The original flowers were red, but many different colours and doubled flowers have been cultivated by plant breeders. A long tube sticks out of the center of the flower with the yellow anthers that contain pollen.

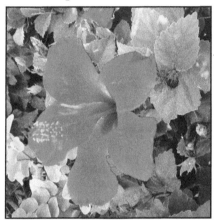

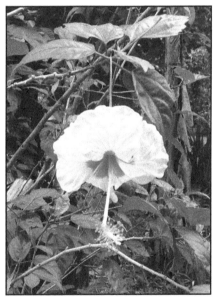

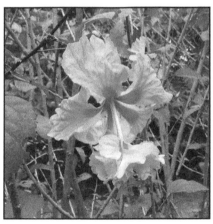

Tea made from hibiscus flowers is used to stop hemorrhages. Tea made from the root is used for contraception. The leaves are made into a hair tonic to stop hair loss and encourage re-growth.

CONVOLVULACEAE

Ipomoea sp.

alepa

Alepa grows as a bush with heart-shaped leaves on branched stems. The yellow flowers have five petals that drop off leaving flat-edged fruits with ten chambers that are used as a stamp to decorate corn biscuits and tortillas.

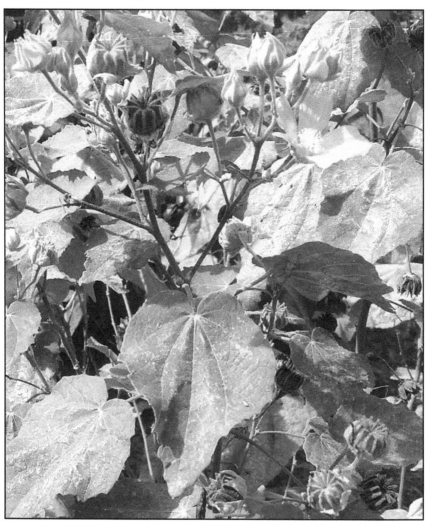

This domesticated plant is becoming rarer and rarer because it is used only by the Maya. Alepa stops hemorrhages by applying the water from boiled leaves directly to the skin. It is also used in holistic baths.

Justicia breviflora (Nees) Rusby

zorillo macho, skunk root, pi' che'

Zorillo macho is an herb with shiny opposite oblong leaves with a central vein and smooth edges. Many small white flowers arise opposite along a long stem.

The leaves of both zorillo plants, when mashed, smell like skunk. Zorillo macho with the bigger leaf is the male. A related species with a smaller leaf is the female called "zorillo hembra." Both are used for the same purposes.

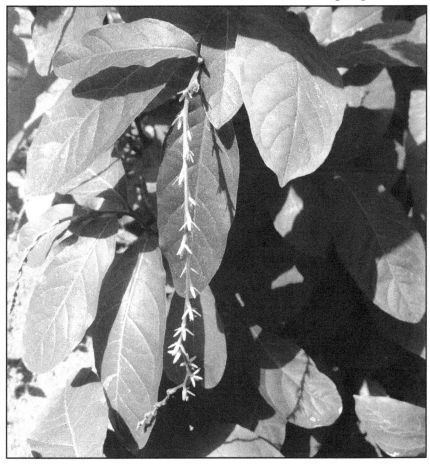

Zorillo leaves are used for purification in baths. Teas from the stems and leaves of this plant for relaxation, stress, insomnia, anxiety relief, can be used. For scabes or rash from poisonwood, apply tea to the lesions or drink the tea. For mild strokes, use the leaves in a bath.

CRASSULACEAE

Kalanchoe pinnata (Lam.) Pers.

siempreviva, life everlasting

Siempreviva is a plant growing to one meter tall. The leaves are waxy light green with violet along the zigzagged edges. New plants are produced from the edges of leaves that drop off. The flowers are papery tubes that hang down, pink at the base and yellow at the end.

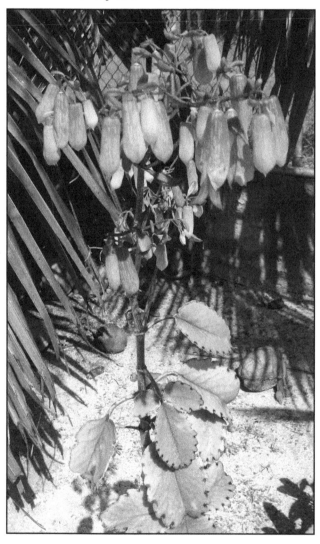

A tincture or ointment can be made from siempreviva leaves to put directly on mumps or inflammed areas.

Lantana camara L.

wild oregano, lantana, ore'go ich che'

Wild oregano is a shrub growing to one meter with prickly stems. The opposite hairy oval leaves have pointed tips and toothed edges. The small flowers are in round clusters that vary from yellow around the outside to red centers, but the colours change as they age.

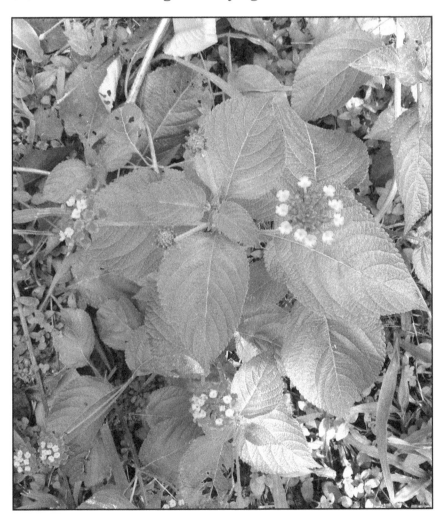

Tea made from wild oregano leaves is used to relieve gastritis because of too much gas. The leaves are also used for baths for thickening of the blood (pasmo).

Lantana sp.

wild grape, oregano

Wild grape grows as a low plant with dark green, thick alternate leaves (8 cm) that have a dull, fuzzy appearance with finely serrated edges. The small lavender flowers develop into bunches of green berries (seeds) that turn lavender when ripe and look like bunches of grapes, which accounts for the common name.

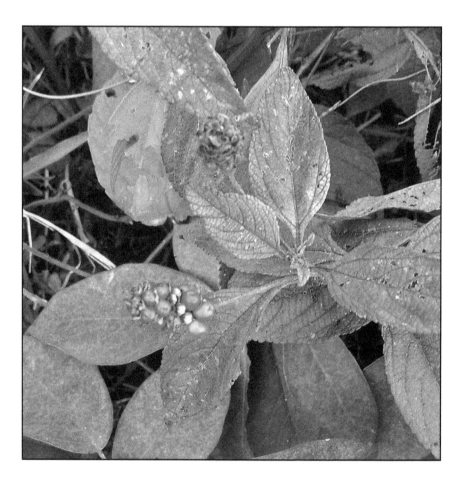

The fruit of this plant is edible. Drink tea made from wild grape leaves every morning before breakfast for arthritis, rheumatism, or other pain. Baths and tinctures made with wild grape leaves can be used to heal pain, arthritis, and rheumatism.

Licania platypus (Hemsl.) Fritsch

monkey apple, sansapote, succotz

Monkey apple grows as a tree with oblong alternate leaves with pointed tips. The large (20 cm) brown-skinned fruit with orange-yellow pulp has a sweet flavor.

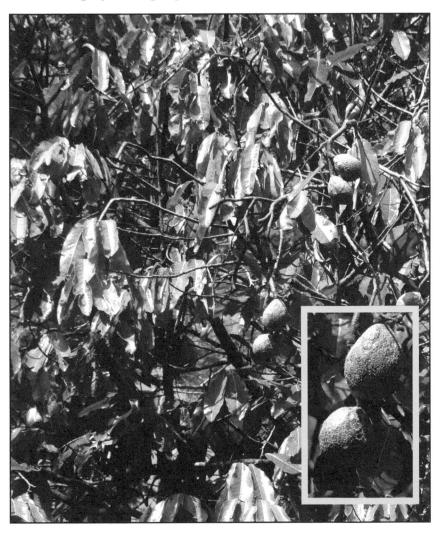

Tea made from monkey apple bark is used for diarrhea and hepatitis, and as a disinfectant. The fruits of this tree are rich in vitamin C.

The village of Succotz is named after the Mayan name of the fruit from this tree (succotz).

Lippia alba (Mill.) N.E. Br. ex Britton & P. Wilson

small oregano, ore'go

Small oregano is a small shrub with slender arching branches. The small opposite leaves (3 cm) are oval with rounded tips and finely serrated edges. The leaves are aromatic when crushed. Small pink flowers are clustered on short stems that come from the same place on the stem as the leaves.

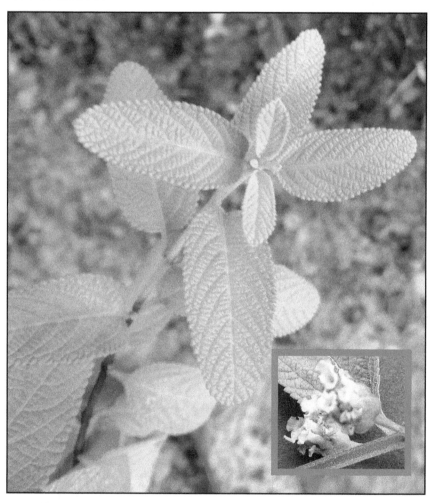

Small oregano leaf tea is used for digestive problems, such as belly-ache or worms. It can also be used as a disinfectant by washing the affected area to heal wounds.

Lippia graveolens Kunth

thick oregano, nuuk lea', Mexican oregano, ore'go

Thick oregano is a shrub with a round shape. The thick leaves have hairs on the top and bottom. Small white flowers are clustered on short stems from where the leaf attaches to the stem.

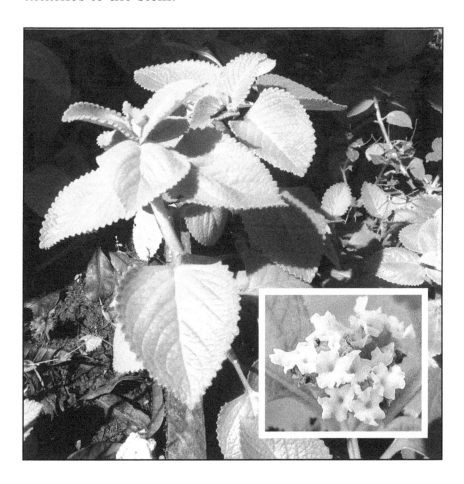

Thick oregano leaves are boiled to use as a disinfectant to dry wounds quickly and as a douche. An oil made with the leaves is used to treat earaches. Freshly mashed leaves can be put on any inflamed area. It is used for paralysis in animals; brush the animal with the shrub and then thrown it away.

Lygodium heterodoxum Kunze
hetero fern

This wild fern likes open areas. They grow like vines hanging onto a tree, but they are ferns because they have fiddleheads that unfurl into leaves. The leaf shape varies from oblong leaves (5 cm) with pointed tips, sometimes with two or more lobes to narrow leaves, also sometimes with lobes.

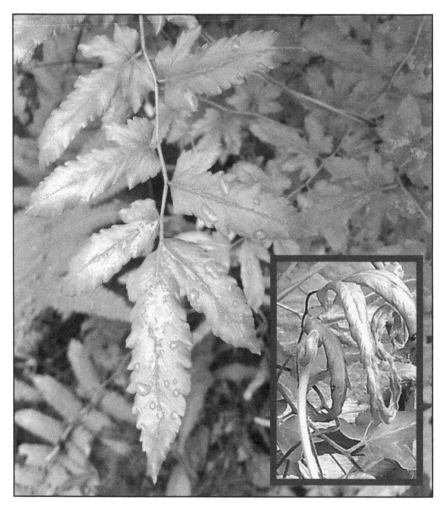

This fern is good for fungus infections and ring worm. The leaves are boiled and made into a tincture. Wash the affected area up to three times every day. This tincture is only for topical use, not to drink.

SCHIZAEACEAE

Lygodium venustum Sw.

alambre, wire wisk, corremiento

This fern has an unusual leaf shape. The long (30 cm) alternate leaves are rounded at the tip and have many small (2 cm) protrusions along the sides. Like other ferns, these leaves unfurl from a fiddlehead. The alambre is considered the male counterpart of the hetero fern.

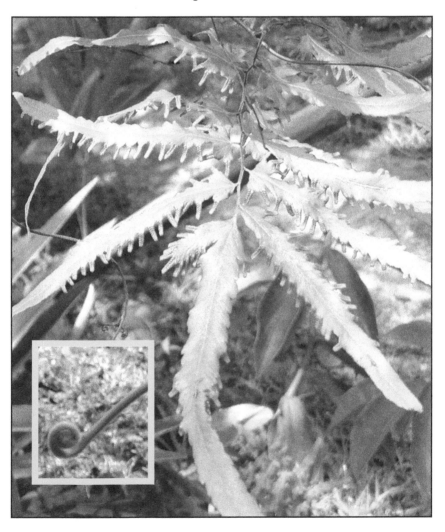

Leaves of this fern are boiled and made into a tincture to treat athlete's foot, or other fungus infections.

ANACARDIACEAE

Mangifera indica L.

mango

Mangos are large, round, full trees with dark green narrow alternate leaves (25 cm) in swirls at the ends of branches. Small yellow flowers are in clusters on branched spikes sticking up from the ends of stems. Mango fruits are popular and sweet. Mango trees bear fruit only once per year.

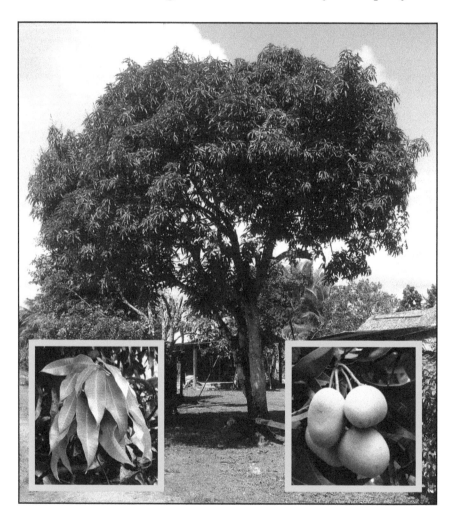

The young leaves are used for teas to prevent coughs. They have a lot of vitamin C. The resin is good for expelling warts and for treating ringworm and leishmaniasis.

Manilkara zapota (L.) P. Royen

chicle, sapodilla, ya'

Chicle is a tree that grows in Belizean forests. It provided a major source of income in northern and western Belize during the early to middle 20th Century. Chicleros collected the sap for a major component of chewing gum until a synthetic alternative was developed. The leaves with pointed tips are clustered at the tips of short stems. The round brown fruit (5 cm diameter) is noticeable because it stays on the tree for 10 months of the year.

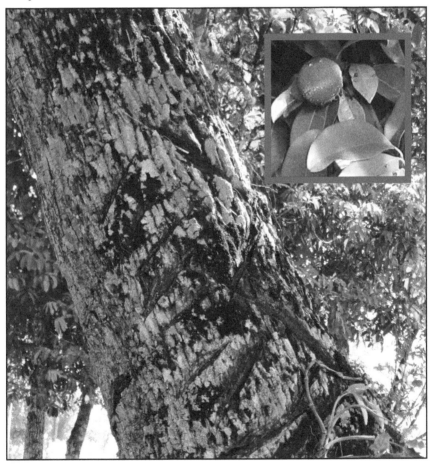

Tea made from chicle bark cleanses the blood and digestion, so it acts like a purge, and can treat diarrhea. It can also be used to wash affected areas with sores as it disinfects and allows them to heal quickly.

FABACEAE : Mimosoideae

Mimosa pudica L.

sensitive plant, mimosa, adormidilla, twelve o'clock, ix mu'tz

Sensitive plants grow even in backyards and roadsides as tall as one meter. When it is touched, the leaves fold up toward each other. The compound, oblong leaves with rounded tips and bases, have pink edges, as many as 25 pairs on a stem. The lilac flowers are balls of little spikes (1 cm diameter).

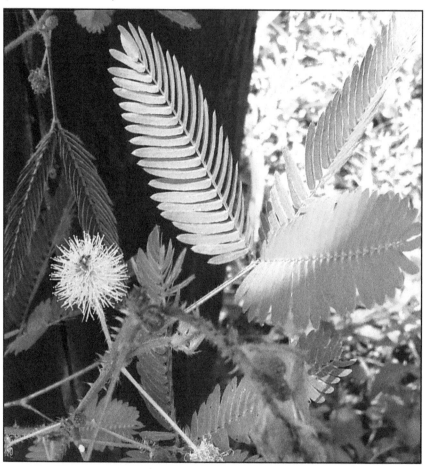

Bathing with sensitive plant leaves can help with sleep problems. Tea made with sensitive plant leaves can also be drunk, but must be used with care because it is strong enough to cause an overdose. Leaves can also placed under the pillow, or the sheet in a baby's bed to help with sleep problems.

Momordica charantia L.

sorosi, ix yamor

Sorosi is a vine with delicate five-lobed leaves each with smaller lobes. The yellow flower has five petals. The bright orange fruit is round with a pointed tip and small thorns on longitudinal ridges.

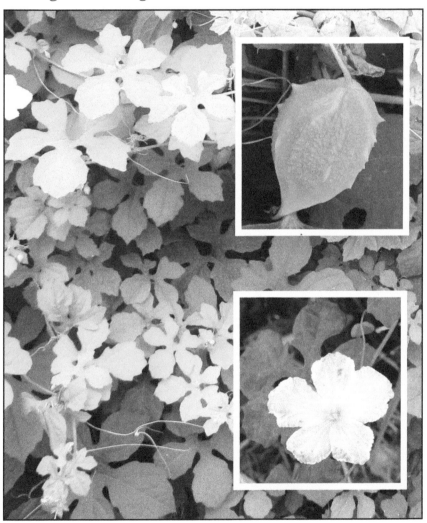

Sorosi is the most commonly used medicinal plant in Belize. Tea made from sorosi leaves and vine cleanses the blood. It is used for cancer, pain, de-worming, and as a tonic.

Morinda citrifolia L.

noni

Noni grows as a small tree. The stiff dark green opposite leaves have prominent veins, smooth edges, and rounded tips. The small white flowers open out of a green cluster, first as tiny tubes, and then open petals. The fleshy yellow fruit is actually a combination of the several fruits developing from the cluster of flowers.

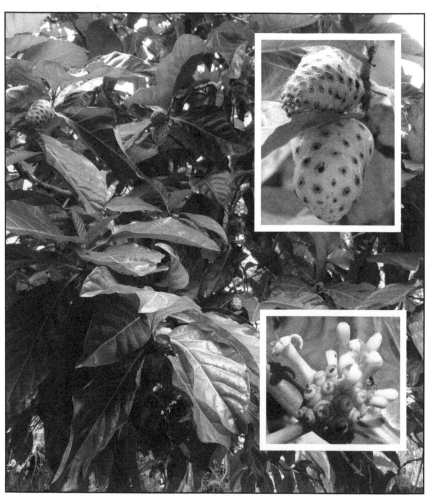

Tea from noni leaves is used to treat AIDS and diabetes. Noni fruit juice is also used for AIDS and for prevention, to keep healthy.

Neurolaena lobata (L.) R. Br. ex Cass.

jackass bitters, tres puntas, mano de lagarto, na' suuon, nuuk suun

Jackass bitters is a shrub that grows throughout Belize along roadsides and in fields. Young leaves are long and slender, but as they mature three points appear, the tip and one on each side. The small yellow flowers are in clusters at the ends of stems.

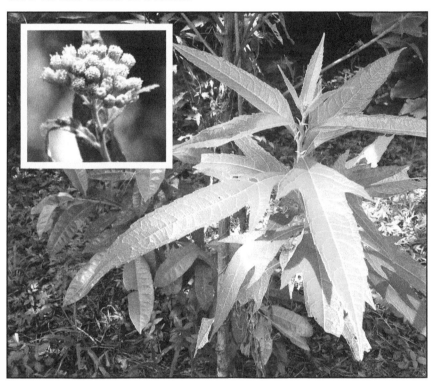

Jackass bitters is one of the most commonly used herbs in Mayan herbal healing. It is boiled and drunk to purify the blood and treat cancer, diabetes, pain, worms, and internal infections. It is used to prevent malaria and to clear a previous malaria infection that continues to reoccur.

Applied to the skin, a tincture made from jackass bitters leaves treats fungal infections, other skin lesions, and acts as a general antibiotic and insect repellent. Traditionally, the Maya drink jackass bitters for a week three times a year to stay in good health and ward off diseases like cancer and diabetes.

Ocimum basilicum L.

basil, albahaca, kekeltun, kakaltun

Basil grows as a small plant with oblong leaves with pointed tips and bases. They grow around a central stem with light green flowers in layers on a stalk at the top of the stem. Basil is recognized by high scent of the leaves and seed pods. It is common in savannahs.

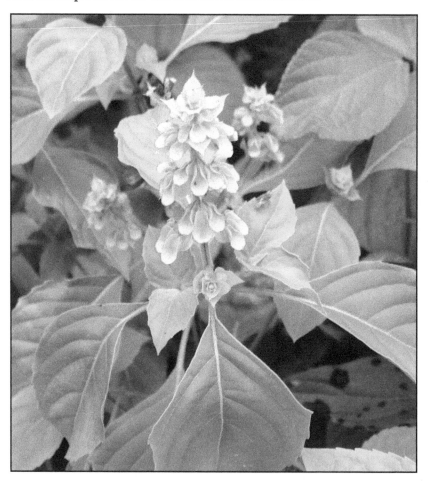

Basil seeds are used to clean the eyes; put a few seeds in eyes before you go to sleep and in the morning, the dirt will come out. Tea made from the leaves is used for urinary and digestive problems, de-worming, and for holistic baths for evil eye and stress. It is a good luck plant to have at the front of your house.

Opuntia cochenillifera (L.) Mill.

prickly pear, nopal, ix placan

Prickly pear is a cactus with thick stems and flat leaves with rounded edges and thorns on the surface. Red flowers grow out of the edge of the leaves.

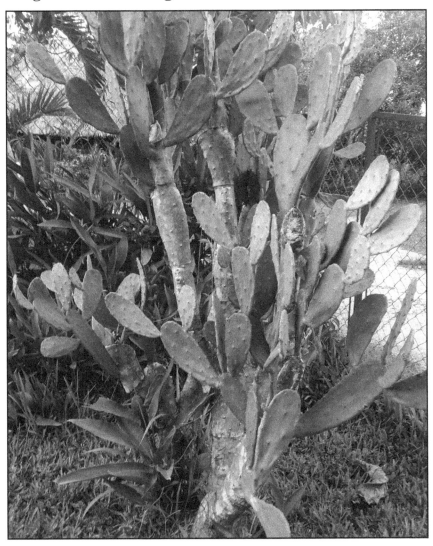

Prickly pear leaf is used as a hair conditioner and to reverse hair loss. The leaf cut in half is used to heal sunburn, other burns, ulcers, and open sores. To treat a headache, put half of a leaf on your head.

Persea Americana Mill.

avocado, pear, oon

Avocados grow as a tall, straight tree. The oblong leaves (8 cm) with rounded tips are in clusters at the ends of branches. The sides of the leaves curl up making a boat that bends toward the tip. The avocado tree bears a delicious, protein-filled fruit once a year from July through September; it is domesticated and grows well throughout Belize.

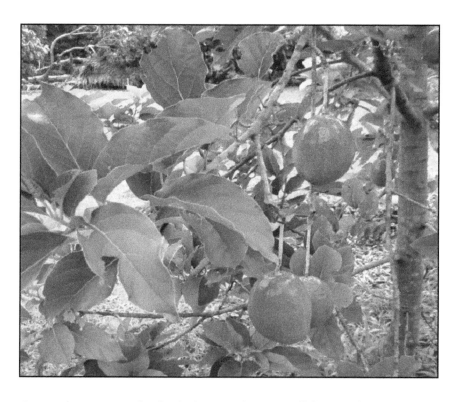

Over-ripe avocado fruit is used a conditioner for dry and damaged hair. Avocado leaves can be boiled for tea that cures hemorrhages such as bruises, and when combined with honey, it forms a cough syrup, which is especially good to treat bad coughs associated with asthma. Make an ointment from the seeds and massage it into joints to treat rheumatism and arthritis. Tea from the bark or seed of the avocado tree can be used as a contraceptive.

Philodendron hederaceum (Jacq.) Schott

mutazai, philodendron

Mutazai is a vine with a small (6 cm) heart-shaped leaf.

Mutazai is used to bathe babies to make their bones stronger so they will walk sooner, but it is poisonous, so it must not be taken internally.

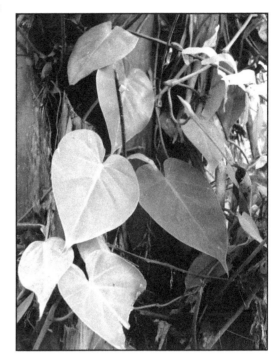

Philodendron sp.

philodrendron

This *Philodrendron* species has a large leaf (30 cm) with prominent veins and smooth edges.

Tinctures made from the leaves of this *Philodrendron* species is used to treat ringworm, athlete's foot, leishmaniasis, and rebellious sores.

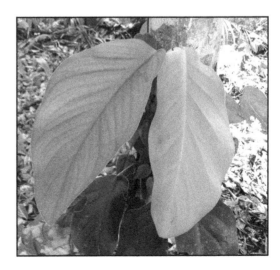

Phlebodium decumanum (Willd.) J. Sm.

calawala, cola de mico

Calawala grows as an epiphyte with hairy roots. The light green leaves are divided into at least nine alternate long, pointed leaflets. The male counterpart of the calawala is cola de mico (p. 143).

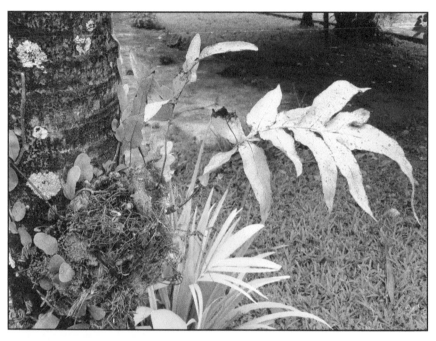

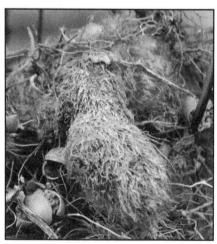

Calawala root tea is used to treat cancer and soaked leaves are a component of hair tonic.

calawala roots

Phyllanthus amarus Schumach. or *Phyllanthus niruri* L.

mallard stone, harry tom, stone breaker

Mallard stone is a small plant growing in yards and other open areas. The tiny oval leaves (5mm) are dark green on the top, but light green on the bottom. Underneath are yellow glands lined up with each pair of leaves. Older stems turn red. Flowers are yellow with a few petals on the stems.

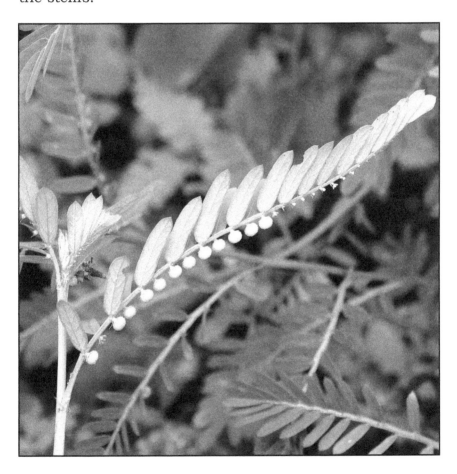

Mallard stone leaves made into a tea are helpful for stomach ulcers and kidney stones. Mallard stone can be used as a holistic bath for evil eye, *mal de ojo*. The structure of the plant is symbolic because the eyes are hiding underneath.

Pimenta dioica (L.) Merr.

allspice, pimienta gorda, naba kuuk

Allspice grows as a medium tall tree in hilly areas, like the Cayo and Toledo Districts. The dark green long (20 cm) leaves, pointed at both ends, grow around the stem. The flowers and fruits develop at the ends of stems as branched structures with small spheres at the end of each branch. The smooth allspice bark is a distinguishing feature.

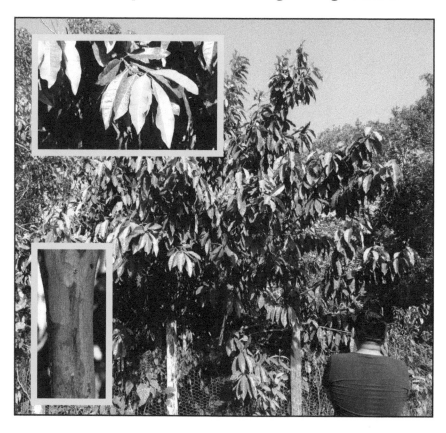

Allspice leaf tea is used to normalize body temperature, so it is good for fever or hot flashes. Allspice leaf tea helps to digest food. The dried seeds can be crushed and boiled in water with salt for belly pain and diarrhea.

Allspice leaves are used in many Mayan sacrificial ceremonies. They are spread on the ground where they chant or do ritual dancing and, as the allspice leaves are crushed, the aroma purifies the area.

PIPERACEAE

Pipers are distinguished by the shapes of their leaves, their flowers, and the scent of their crushed leaves. Pipers are sacred to the Maya, an important component of holistic baths.

Leaves from any piper can be boiled or crushed and then applied on the head to treat headaches. Piper leaves can be chewed to strengthen teeth and gums. Piper leaves can also be used to relax and purify the mind and body. The leaves of all pipers are used in baths for rheumatism, arthritis, pain, and swellings. They can also be used for minor strokes and paralysis. The root of any piper can be used for snakebites.

There are many piper species. We have photographs of nine of the pipers found in Belize. We have specifically identified three, but for others we do not know the scientific name. Because nine species are used for a holistic bath, it is important to recognize many different piper species.

PIPERACEAE

Piper peltatum

peltatum piper

The leaves of this piper are the same size as cowfoot (40 cm) except the stem of this piper is attached under the leaf about one-quarter of the way to the tip, and the leaves are wrinkled. The flowers are five or six short white spikes sticking up clustered at the end of a stem. The Maya believe this particular plant is the male companion to cowfoot. If you crush the leaf, it doesn't have a minty or licorice scent.

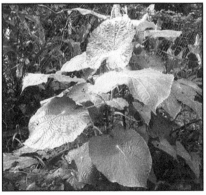 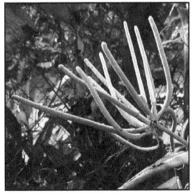

In addition to its other uses as a piper, tea made from this piper is good for allergies and for internal cleansing after having given birth.

Piper auritum Kunth

cowfoot, obel

Cowfoot is a shrub with large, heart-shaped leaves (40 cm) with one tall white spike (20 cm) sticking up at the base of the leaf. The leaves have a pleasant licorice or anise smell when crushed. A relative of the black pepper used to spice foods, cowfoot grows about seven meters high, but only where light is available.

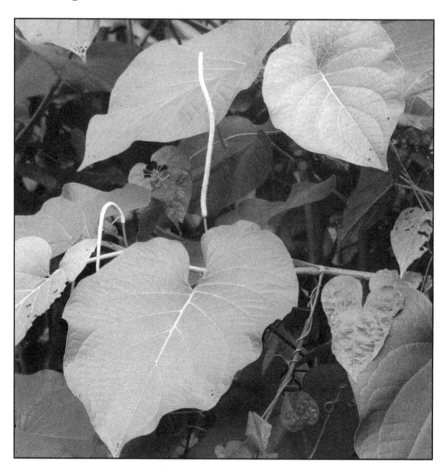

Cowfoot leaves are used in holistic baths and to make tea to treat sprains, strains, inflammation, bruises, pain, and toothaches. Cowfoot has also been reported to treat fertility problems. The soft tip of the stem on the top is edible and is a de-wormer.

Piper jacquemontianum Kunth

cordoncillo, Spanish elder, buttonwood, pu' chuch

Cordoncillo is in the piper family, one of the most abundant families in Central and South America. Similar to cowfoot (*Piper auritum*), they are distinguished by the shape of the leaves. Cordoncillo leaf is elongated and has a pointed tip and rounded base, while cowfoot is heart-shaped. The flower of cordoncillo is shorter (10 cm) than cowfoot and each leaf has two or three.

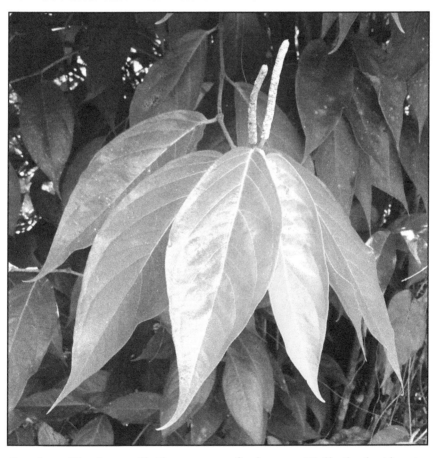

Cordoncillo has all the uses of pipers: Holistic baths to relax and purify the mind and body, baths for rheumatism, arthritis, pains, swellings, minor strokes and paralysis. Leaves can be applied to the head to treat headaches, or chewed to strengthen teeth and gums. The roots can be used for snakebites.

Piper sp.

This piper has an oval leaf with a long pointed tip. Several white flowers (10 cm) arise out of the stem.

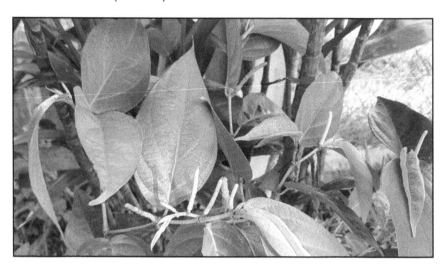

Piper sp.

This piper leaf (25 cm) has a rounded base and pointed tip. Additional veins radiate from the central vein.

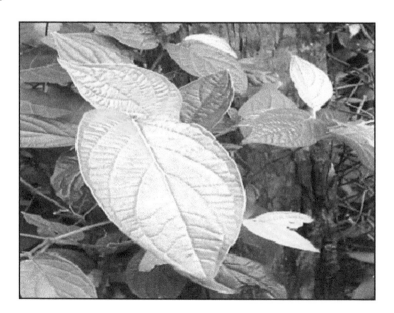

Piper sp.

The leaf of this piper (*right*) has two equal lobes, each pointed at the tip. The flower is two or three white spikes that lay across the base of the leaf.

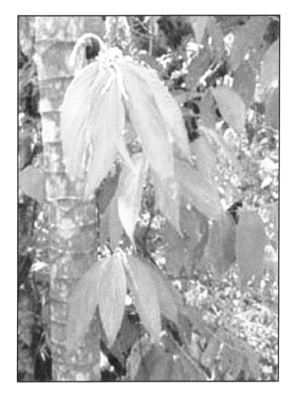

Piper sp.

This piper (*below*) has a small leaf (12 cm) with a rounded base and pointed tip.

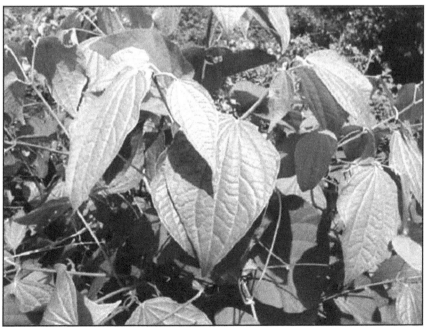

Piper sp.

The dark green leaves (10 cm) of this piper (*right*) are rounded with a finely pointed tip. The long white flowers droop. The veins parallel the edge of the leaf.

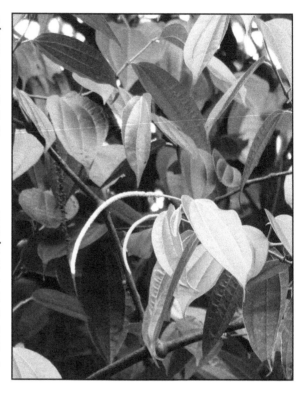

Piper sp.

This piper (*below*) has a small (10 cm) oblong leaf with a blunt tip, shiny surface, and smooth edges. The white flowers stick up at the node and some break open.

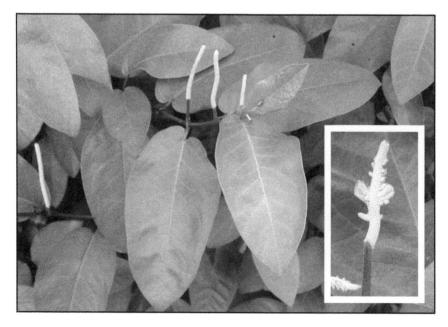

Pluchea carolinensis (Jacq.) G. Don

cha'al che', santa maria, cough bush, cure-for-all, ix cha'al che'

Cha'al che' is a wild shrub that grows mainly in open areas. The stems are hairy and the oval leaves are hairy on top with a pointed tip. The leaves have a scent like mint. It has pale purple flowers.

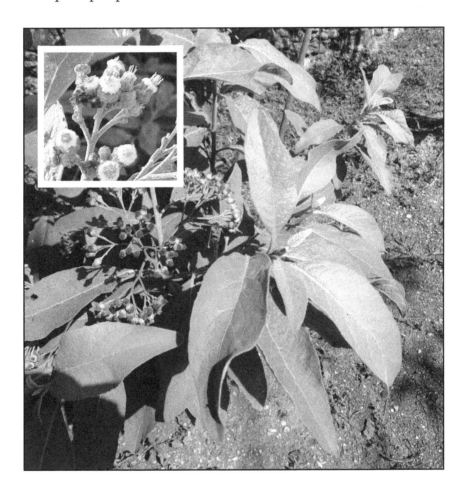

The leaves of cha'al che' are boiled to make a tea, which is used after birthing to flush out the impurities and heal the womb faster. The tea is also used for treating menstrual cramps and for coughs. The resin from the cut stem is used to treat skin lesions such as wounds, warts, ringworm, and leishmanaisis.

ASTERCEAE

Porophyllum punctatum (Mill.) S.F. Blake
ma'mu'kal, hierba de piojillo, squirrel's tail, tah tai'i

Ma'mu'kal is a small plant with dark stems and oppo-site small, rounded leaves with three slight indentations. When you crush the leaves, they stink like skunk, which accounts for the Spanish name, *piojillo*, which means "stink."

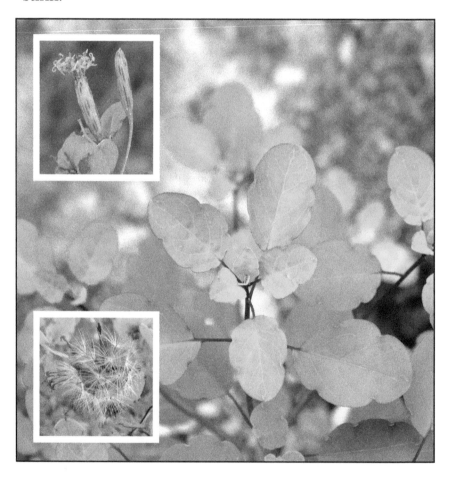

Ma'mu'kal is an energy booster for those who have lost their strength through strokes. It is used in holistic baths and oils and for cleansing to expel sickness around you.

PORTULACACEAE

Portulaca oleracea L.

hierba buena, verdolaga

Hierba buena spreads on the ground as a mat. The fleshy alternate leaves (5 cm) are oval and rounded at the tip. The flowers (3 cm across) are yellow.

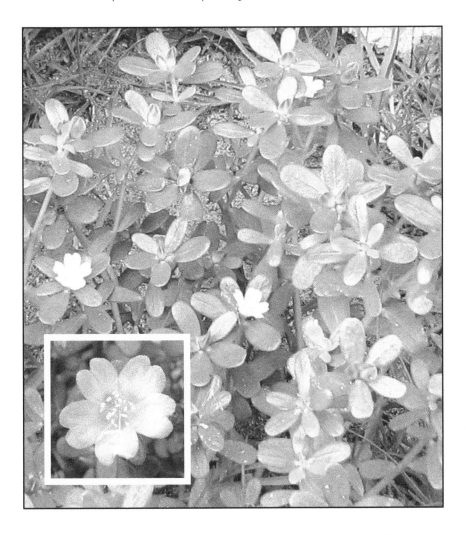

Hierba buena leaves are used to make a tea to decrease the menstrual flow for women. The leaves are also used to treat nightmares. They are spread under the pillow or sheet to make sweet dreams.

VERBENACEAE

Priva lappulacea (L.) Pers.

mosote, cat's tongue, ix tabay, pech ma'am

Mosote is a small plant with opposite leaves (10 cm long) that are oval with a pointed tip and toothed edges. The tiny tubular flowers are pale blue to violet. The outside of the tiny nut fruits (3 mm) is covered with hooked hairs that cling to clothing.

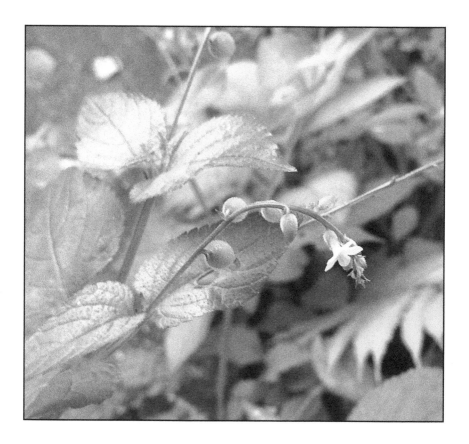

Tea from mosote stem and juice from the leaves expell kidney and gall bladder stones.

Protium copal (Schltdl. & Cham.) Engl.

copal, pom

Copal grows as a tall tree in the riverine forests of Belize. The distinctive bark has white blotchy spots on the brown background. The oval leaves (10 cm) have slightly pointed tips. The small nuts are oblong with rounded points on one end.

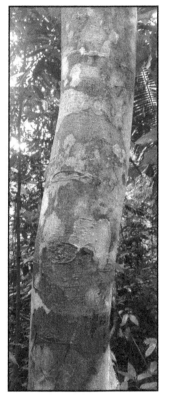
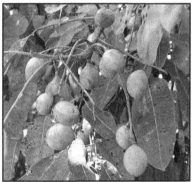
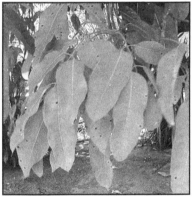

Copal is very significant to the Maya. The tree contains resin, which is extracted and burned as incense in all ceremonies, such as, *primisias* of purification, thanksgiving, and supplication. Ceremonies are performed where copal incense is burned in the milpas before planting and harvesting.

The smell of the resin removes a headache and heals hemorrhages of the nose. Copal is used in the smudge (*p. 17*), by itself only if it is an offering, mass or christening, but for cleansing and purification, it is combined with other plants.

MYRTACEAE

Psidium guajava L.

guava, guyaba, p'tah

Guava is a wild, adaptable tree that can grow in many places, from forests to streambeds to backyards. The opposite oval leaves (15 cm long by 5 cm wide) have rounded tips and smooth edges. The stems are smooth. The white fragrant flowers (1.5 cm) have petals and fine white spikes. The green round fruit (3 cm) turns yellow when ripe. It is entirely edible and rich in vitamin C.

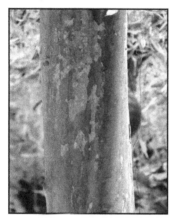 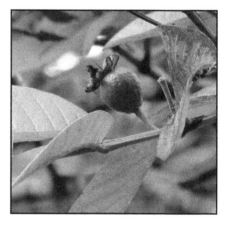

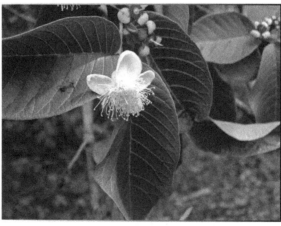

Guava bark is used to treat diarrhea. The boiled leaves are used as a douche. Just after giving birth, women are washed with the boiled leaves to clean them faster, dry quicker, prevent infection, reduce inflammation and release pain. Boiled leaves can also be used as a disinfectant to wash sores or wounds.

SIMAROUBACEAE

Quassia amara L.

palo de hombre

Palo de hombre grows as a tree with striking red flowers and berries throughout the year. The stem looks like a narrow leaf with a thick red vein running down the center and narrow green edges. Leaves come out of nodes in the stems, either two on either side, or one at the end. The long (25 cm) leaves are pointed at both ends and droopy. The red flowers are on red branching stems and start as small red balls at the end of a short stem developing gradually into long tubes (5 cm). The fruit is a round red berry, the same colour as the flowers and their branching stems.

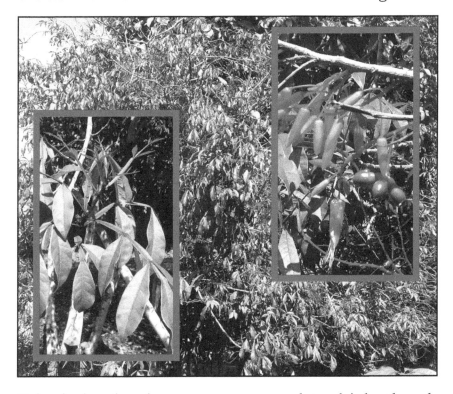

Palo de hombre leaves are very good to drink, though bitter. Tea made from either the leaves or the stem can be used to purify the body and treat dehydration, indigestion, infertility, pain, and worms. It strengthens the blood against diseases, especially AIDS, diabetes and malaria. If anemic, palo de hombre strengthens blood. The leaves can be pulverized to treat cuts and sores.

Ricinus communis L.

castor oil plant, castor bean, higuerilla, aceite ko'och

Castor oil plant is a wild shrub found mainly in the higher elevations of the Cayo or Toledo districts. The large (20 cm or more) alternate leaves have five to seven lobes with narrow tips and serrated edges. The fruits are spiny brown capsules that contain shiny black seeds.

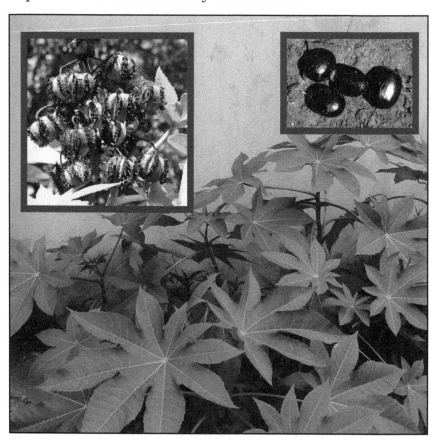

Except for the oil from seeds, the castor oil plant is poisonous, and should not be taken internally. The leaves are used to treat migraine headaches either by boiling and massaging onto the head or by wrapping the uncooked leaves around the head. This also helps to reduce a high fever.

The oil from ground seeds is used as a laxative and as a purge, one tablespoon at a time.

Ruta chalepensis L.

rudah, common rue

Rudah is a small plant with grayish green leaves. The delicate oblong leaves have rounded tips and narrowed bases.

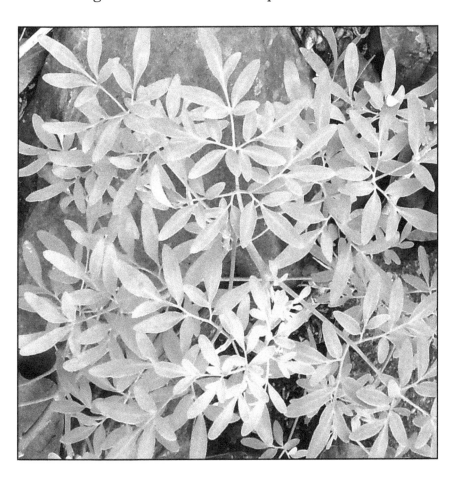

Rudah is a good luck plant for the Maya. It is a domesticated plant. It is used for holistic baths to remove bad spirits or bad luck around. It is used to treat epileptics and unexplained fainting spells. Mashed leaves are soaked in a glass of water for half an hour, which is strained for drinking. Use the same mash to bless a business by sprinkling it around.

Sansevieria hyacinthoides (L.) Druce

mother-in-law tongue

Mother-in-law tongue is a small plant with no stems. The long (50 cm) stiff erect leaves are marbled grey or have faintly mottled bands waving across the leaves. The greenish white, tubular flowers (60 cm tall) are in clusters of three to five along stems that rise from the base at the end of rainy season. The fruits are small berries.

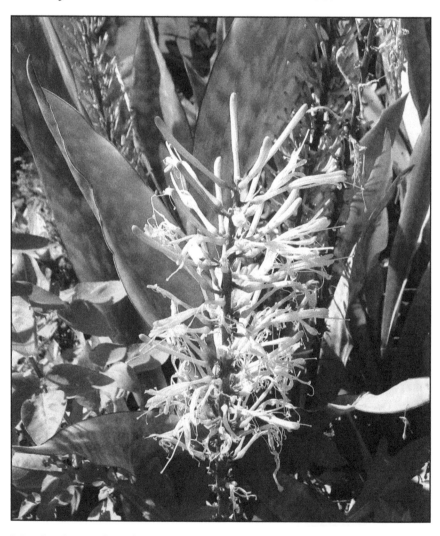

Mashed mother-in-law tongue leaves made into a poulstice are used to treat snakebites.

FABACEAE: Caesalpinioideae

Senna alata (L.) Roxb.

piss-a-bed, candle bush, ix bra' haj

Piss-a-bed grows as a small tree. The compound leaves have ten to twelve pairs of oblong leaflets (5 cm) with wide rounded tips and narrow bases. The spikey flowers are yellow.

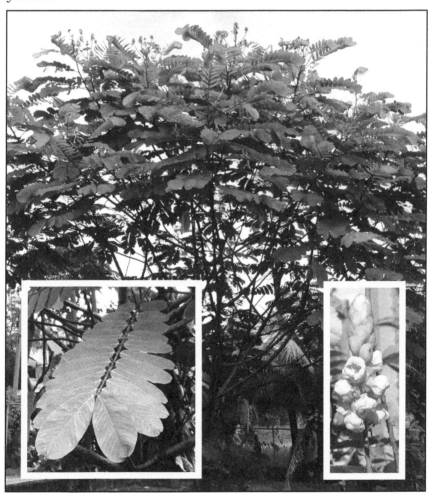

Piss-a-bed leaf tea is very good for a bladder infection. It holds your urine and strengthens the bladder, so piss-a-bed is good to treat bed-wetting. Those with diabetes should take a cup of piss-a-bed tea a day. Tea from the root can be taken for hepatitis. You can also bathe with the leaves for hepatitis.

FABACEAE: Caesalpinioideae

Senna occidentalis (L.) Link

frijolillo

Frijolillo is a shrub with opposite leaves with pointed tips. The leaves at the top of the stem are longest with each leaf shorter to the base of the stem. Friolillo has yellow flowers and red beans on stems. This domesticated plant is common in backyards of the Cayo and Toledo districts.

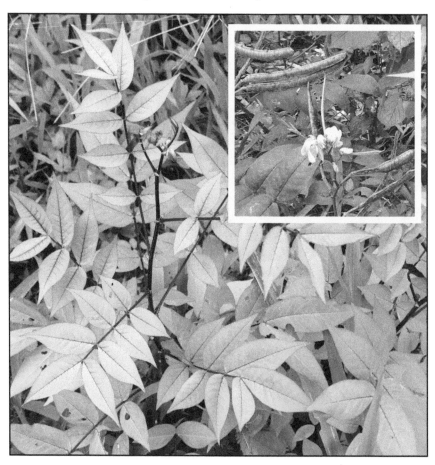

Frijolillo leaves are poisonous to livestock. They can be used as an antiseptic to clean wounds. Oil made from the boiled leaves can be rubbed on the chest to treat fever, asthma, cough, and cold. Frijolillo is used in holistic baths. When children are stubborn and won't listen, pass a friolillo branch over them, and throw it into the river. It can be used for cleansing, along with prayers.

Sida acuta Burm. F.

malva, chichibeh

Malva is a small plant with alternate dark green leaves with pointed tips and serrated edges. The small, rose-like yellow flower opens out of a round green structure on the end of a short stem with each leaf stem.

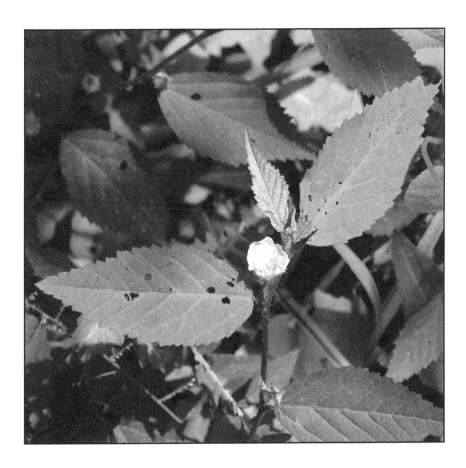

Malva root tea is used to treat bladder infections and stoppage of urine. Malva is used to clean the house, both sweeping and spiritually. When you squeeze the leaf, it is sticky. That sticky substance is used to stop hair loss and to regrow hair. It is used for paralysis in animals; brush the animal with the shrub and then thrown it away.

Simarouba glauca DC.

negrito, dysentery bark

Negrito grows into a tall tree in Belizean riverine forests. The compound leaf is composed of ten to twelve leathery leaflets that are dark green on the top and pale on the bottom. The sweet, black fruits account for the name.

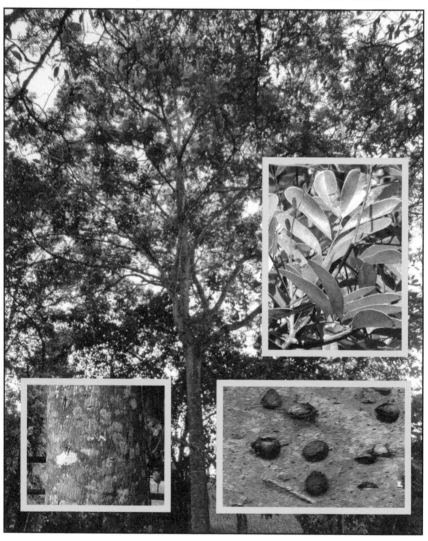

For dysentery and infections in digestive system, tea made from negrito bark acts as a disinfectant.

Sphagneticola trilobata (L.) Pruski

rabbit's paw, u'moch atu'rich, ujanal atu'rich

Rabbit's paw is a dense plant that creeps along the ground and also climbs fences. The bright green opposite leaves are lobed (usually three lobes) with serrated edges. The yellow flowers are daisy-like with narrow petals (3 cm).

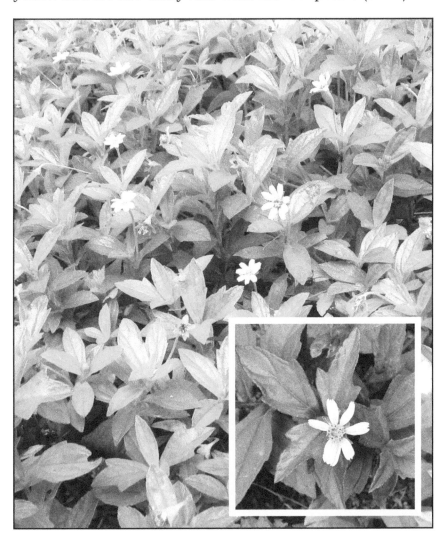

Rabbit's paw is good for sinus, cough, and cold. Make ointment from the leaves and rub it on the forehead, or drink it as a tea.

Spigelia anthelmia L.

worm bush, pinkroot

Worm bush grows on a single stem (30 cm). The opposite leaves are clustered at the top of the stem. They have smooth edges and a long pointed tip. The pink five-lobed flowers (1 cm) are lined up along on a long spike.

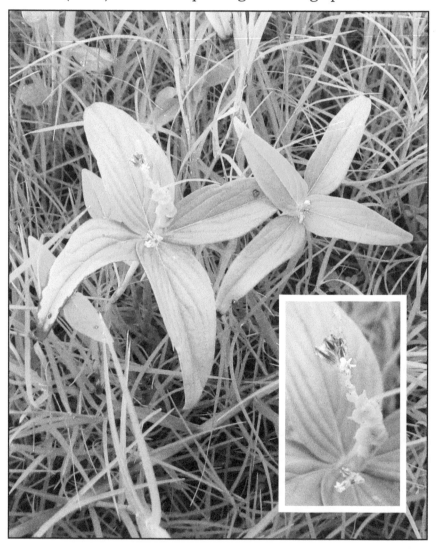

When off balance, drink tea made from worm bush leaves or bathe with it. The tea is also used as a dewormer, which accounts for the name.

Spondias mombin L.

golden plum, a'bül po'ok'oc

Golden plum grows into a large tree with opposite leaves rounded at the base with pointed tips. The small plum fruit grows on branched stems and is golden when ripe. It has a slightly nobby surface. The gray bark is smooth with slight striations.

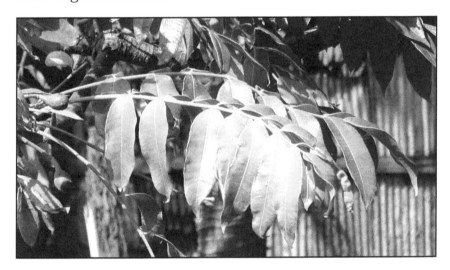

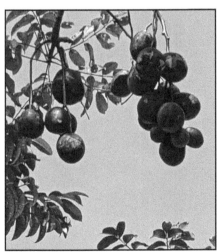
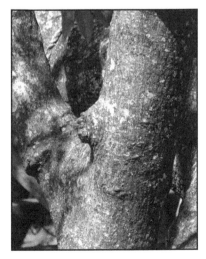

The golden plum resin from the stem or fruit is used as a disinfectant in wounds, ulcers, warts, and leishmaniasis.

NACARDIACEAE

Spondias purpurea L.

may plum, jocote, a'bül

May plum grows to a large tree with compound leaves that are composed of 13 small (8 cm) light green opposite leaflets. The small green plums turn red when ripe and grow right on the branches.

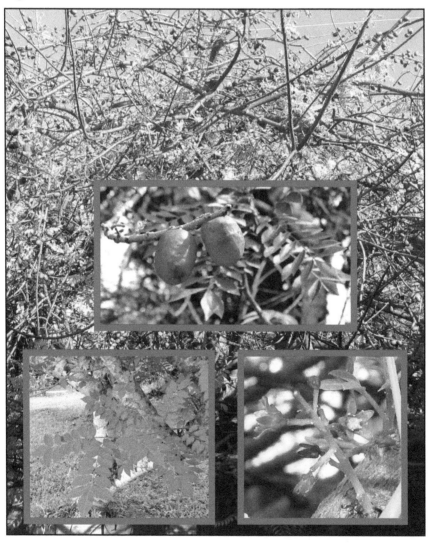

Bathing in tea from the leaves or the bark of may plum is used to treat rashes from allergy or infection. It is a disinfectant for wounds, and helps them to heal quickly.

ANACARDIACEAE

Spondias radlkoferi Donn. Sm.
hog plum, huhub, po'ok'oc

Hog plum grows into a large tree. The stems unfurl like a fern with shiny immature leaves. Mature leaves are oblong with an elongated pointed tip. The bark of a mature tree is rough with vertical troughs. When trees are small, the buds can be eaten raw and are a rich source of vitamin C. This tree bears a plum-like fruit that is edible, but not particularly tasty.

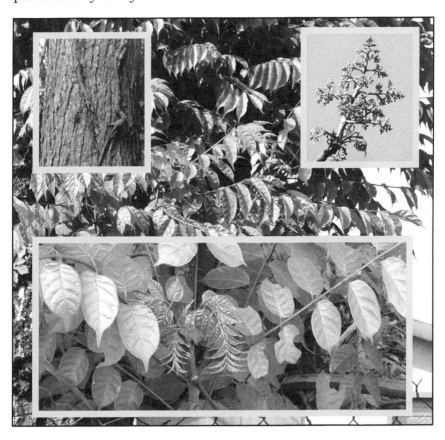

Hog plum leaf tea is very strong, like an antibiotic, so it is used in a bath as a disinfectant for wounds and in general hygienic cleansing. It is excellent for drying cuts and wounds, for skin rashes from allergies, and for skin cancer. Tea made from leaves is used for infection and pain in the womb, fibroma, and cysts.

VERBENACEAE

Stachytarpheta cayennensis (Rich.) Vahl

verbena, vervain, cot-acam, xhi'ic ku'tz

Verbena grows tall (3 m) on a single central stem. The opposite leaves are oval with slightly pointed tips, rounded bases and rough top surfaces. The small lavender flowers (1 cm) are clustered on stems that grow out of the same node as the leaves.

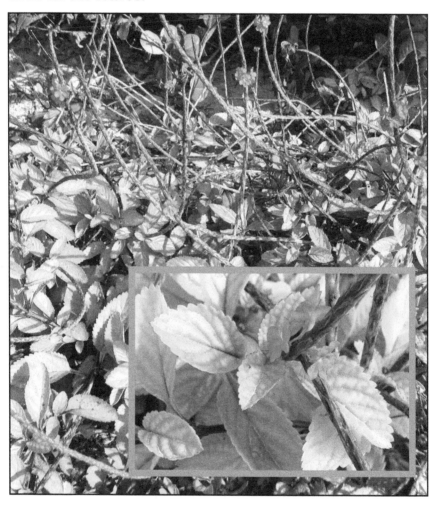

Verbena leaves are used to make a cough syrup. To cure a headache, the leaves can be soaked in water for about half an hour and then washed on the head. Tea made from the roots are good for urinary infection and to level hormones to treat menopause.

APOCYNACEAE

Stemmadenia donnell-smithii (Rose) Woodson

glue tree, horse balls, huevo de caballo, cojoton, p'a tzi'min

Glue tree grows to a medium-sized tree with light green leaves pointed at both ends. The small (2 cm) white flowers have swirled petals. The fruit develops into pairs of large (8 cm) brown oblong balls, giving it the nickname, "horse balls."

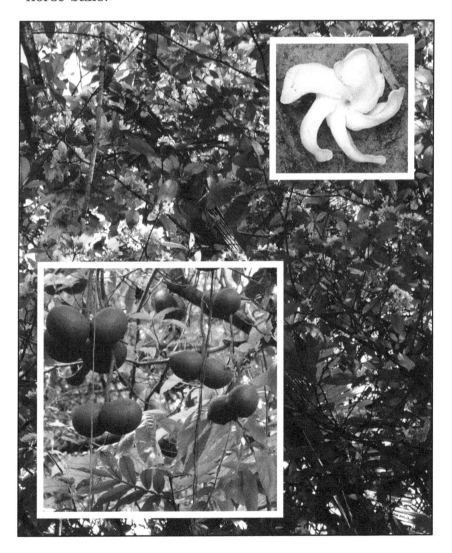

The resin in the stem, branches, leaves, and fruit is glue-like. Botfly larvae can be extracted with this glue.

COMBRETACEAE

Terminalia catappa L.

hamans, Indian almond

This adaptable large evergreen tree branches horizontally, giving it a layered look and makes it popular as a shade tree. The large leathery oval dark green leaves become reddish before dropping. The fleshy oval fruit has an oval nut with a seed inside.

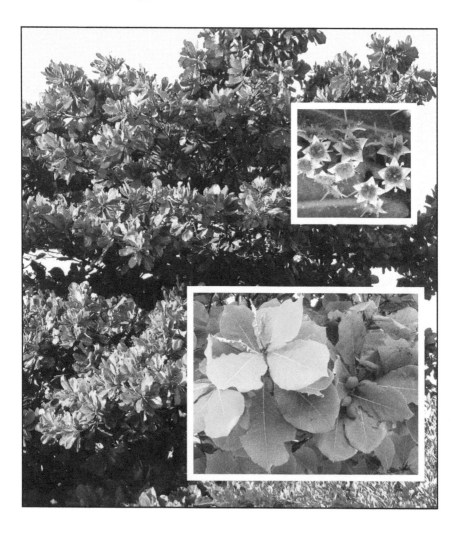

Hamans leaves can be chopped to make a tea that is used to normalize blood pressure and to burn fat to reduce the belly.

Tetragastris panamensis (Engl.) Kuntze

red incense, croton, red copal

Red incense grows into a tall tree with opposite slender leaves (20 cm long) with smooth edges and long points at the tips.

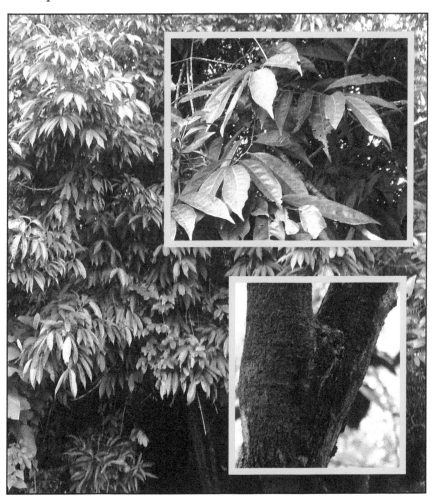

Red incense is a sacred tree for the Maya. Incense from this tree is burned for baptisms and weddings. To get the red incense resin, tap the tree as for copal. The leaves are good for holistic baths. The resin is good for leishmanaisis and removing warts.

MALVACEAE

Theobroma cacao L.

cacao, cocoa, ku' ku'

Cacao grows as a small tree, especially in the shade. The leaves (25 cm) are long ovals pointed at both ends. New leaves at the top are droopy and reddish. As they mature, the leaves become shiny green and more stiff. Tiny white flowers with red anthers arise from the trunk or stems. The oblong fruit is about the same size as the leaves, with distinct ridges. Fruits are light green, turning yellow, orange, or pink when ripe. They grow out of the stem or trunk.

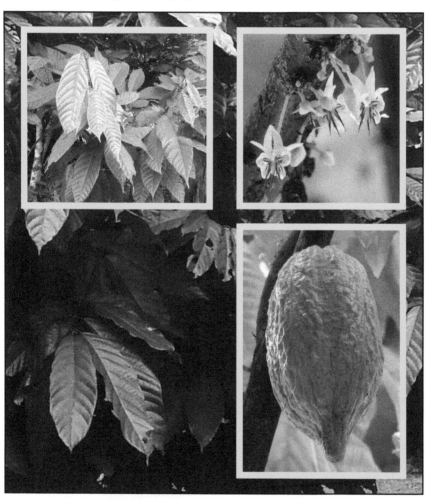

Young cacao leaves are used for hair loss; soak and use as a conditioner; rinse with it; and leave it to dry.

Tradescantia spathacea Sw.

Moses-in-the-cradle, Moses-in-the-boat, spiderwort

Moses-in-the-cradle grows to 30 centimeters tall. The stem is so short that the leaves seem to come out in a circle from the ground. The fleshy leaves are green with light green stripes on the top and purple on the underside. The white flowers with three-lobed petals sit in a purple boat in the center of the circle of leaves.

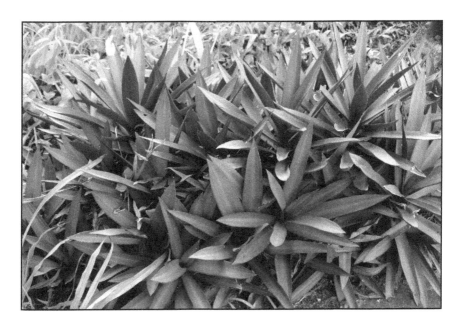

Moses-in-the-cradle leaves are prepared in oil or ointment to apply every day to make scars disappear.

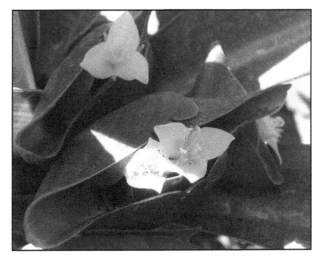

VERBENACEAE

Vitex gaumeri Greenm.

yaxnik

Yaxnik grows as a medium-sized tree with several oval leaves growing around each stem and many branched lavender flowers on separate stems.

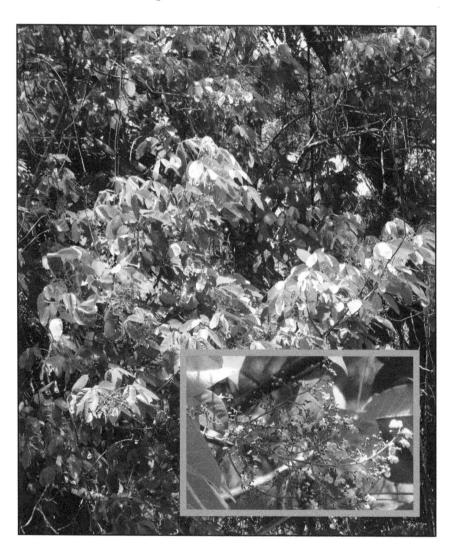

The boiled bark of yaxnik is used to treat leishmaniasis and especially good for rebellious sores that don't want to heal and for skin cancer.

Vochysia hondurensis Sprague
yemeri, white mahogany, sa' wan

Yemeri grows into very tall, straight trees. The leaves are oval, pointed at both ends. Yemeri trees are very notice-able on hillsides in March and April because of their bright yellow flowers. They bear a small light green fruit.

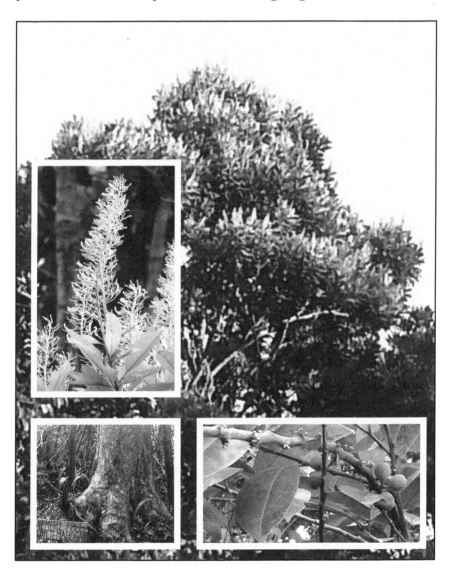

Boiled yemeri bark is used for fungus and leishmaniasis.

GRAMINEAE

Zea mays L.

corn, maize, ix shim (dry corn), mun nal, mun nil (young corn)

Corn grows on a single stalk with long leaves (50 cm). Ears grow out of the stalk inside husks with silk.

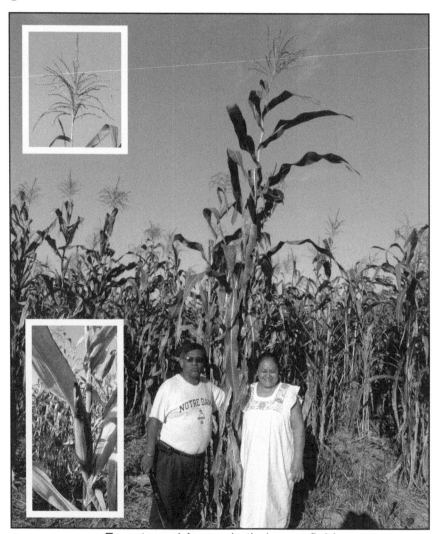

Ernesto and Aurora in their corn field

Boiled silk from either young or dry corn is used to treat kidney stones and urinary infections. A powder can be made from young corn to use with rashes, especially heat rash. After cooking corn with limestone, the water can be used to wash a mother's breast and make the milk flow.

Zingiber officinale Roscoe
ginger, ehimbre

Ginger grows as a low plant with long, narrow, alternate leaves (15 cm).

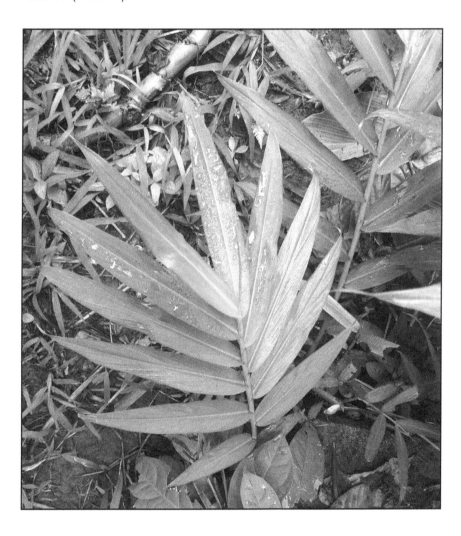

The Maya extract the root of this plant to make a drink with it. The tea is made from mashed ginger roots. The tea is good for everyday consumption and overall health. It is very good for stomach and gas pains. It is also works as a de-wormer and throat disinfectant, and for cold, cough, fever, and general health.

Scientifically Unidentified Plants

acaliptus, keletus, k'eletush, k'le'tux

Acaliptus is a shrub with alternate narrow leaves with long points at the tip, pointed at the stem, and very finely serrated edges. This plant is recognized by short spikes on the underside of the stem.

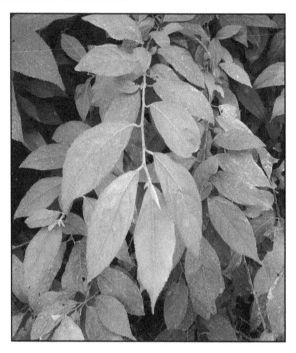

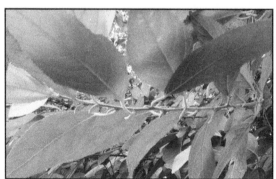

Acaliptus is used similar to stitches. Ground-up leaves stop bleeding when they are placed on the wounded area. They stick to the wound until the leaves dry. When they fall off, it means the wound is healed.

beneno xut

Beneno xut grows on tall thick stems with opposite shiny green leaves pointed at both ends. Several round green fruits grow on short stems out of the same nodes as the leaves.

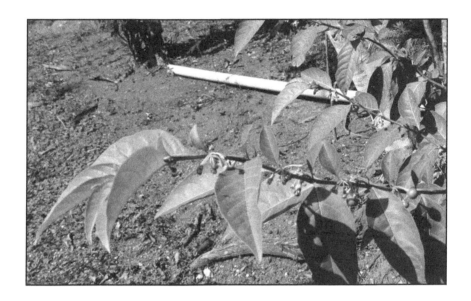

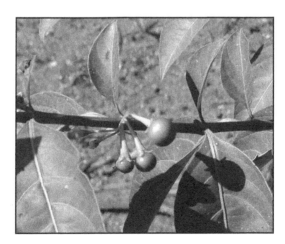

Beneno xut is used in insect repellent.

bob

Bob grows to a large tree with large (35 cm) leaves with prominent veins giving a wrinkled appearance growing on thick stems. The bark is smooth white when young, turning gray in older trees.

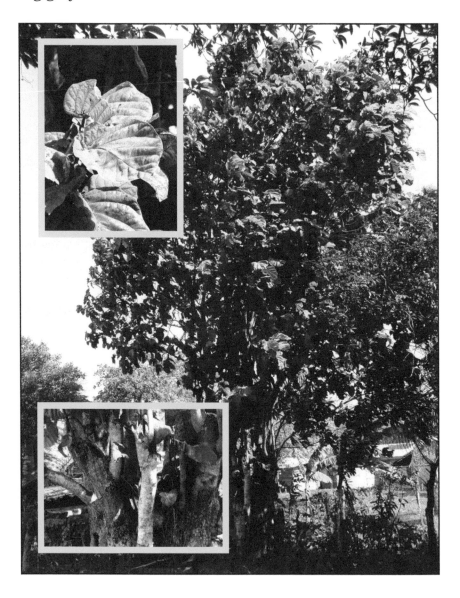

Tea from the leaves of bob is used for arthritis.

cola de mico

This fern has a long compound leaf with as many as 50 pairs of leaflets, which are shorter at the tip, but gradually gain their full length of 10 cm. Each leaflet has a long pointed tip. This compound leaf unfurls from a fiddlehead. Cola de mico is the male counterpart of calawala (*p.102*), but doesn't have the hairy roots of calawala, its female counterpart.

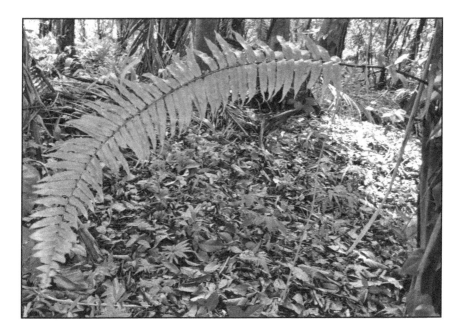

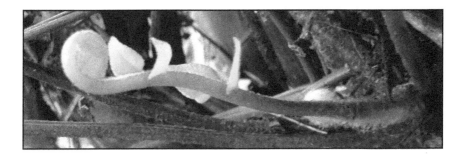

The leaves of cola de mico are ground and made into an oil to be used as a hair conditioner.

corazon, hierba preniada

Corazon is a vine that spreads on fences. The heart-shaped leaves are spongy. The small yellow flowers hang down in a cluster below a stack of thick light green petals.

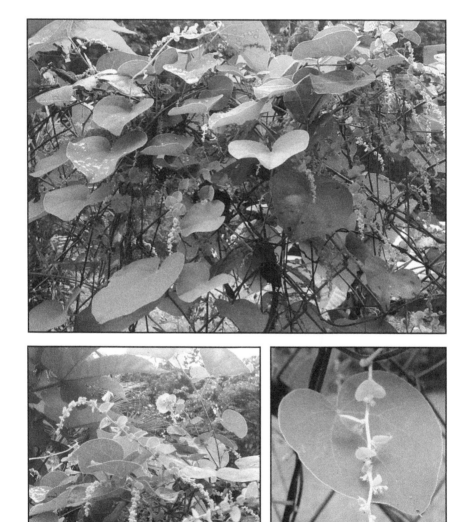

Washing the area with corazon leaf tea is good for infections that are serious like gangrene.

horse bush

Horse bush, so-called because horses like to eat it, is a low herb with grayish leaves that have many lobes and scalloped edges. The small white flowers are on branched stems.

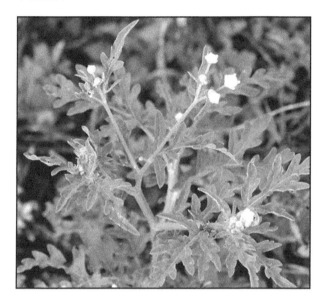

Tea made from horse bush leaves is used to treat scabes, and as an insect repellent.

Washing with the tea removes swelling.

ho'tz

Ho'tz is a thick stalk with many narrow (5mm wide by 10 cm long) leaves with pointed tips growing opposite around the stalk.

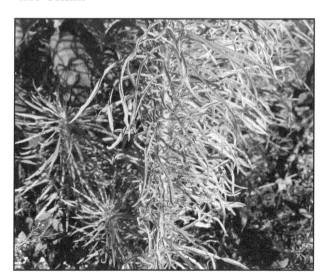

Ho'tz leaf tea is used to treat headaches.

ix cat, wild cucumber

Ix cat grows as a tree with dark shaggy bark and small oval leaves growing three on a stem. The fruits are elongated light green with longitudinal troughs.

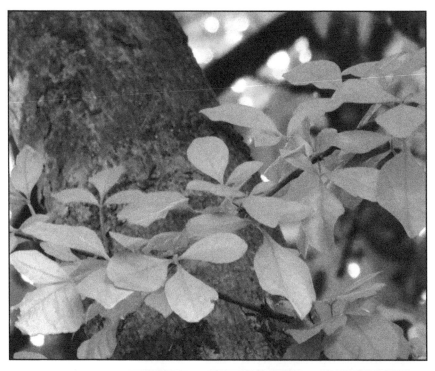

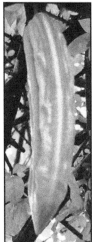
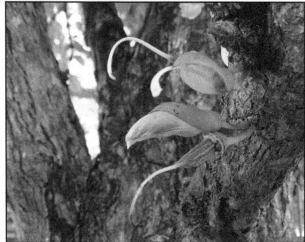

Ix cat bark tea is used as a blood purifier and to treat depression, worry and anxiety.

ix tuc'ulil

Ix tuc'ulil grows as a tree with dark green oblong opposite leaves with smooth edges and rounded tips. Pinkish flowers are spikes growing between the two leaves at the end of the stem.

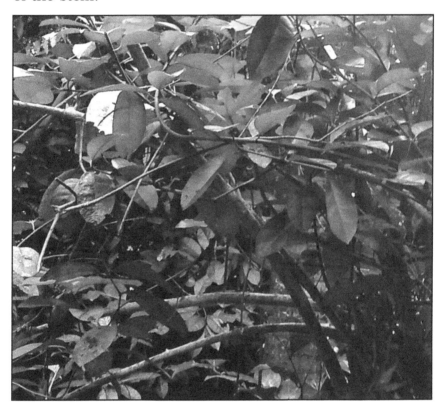

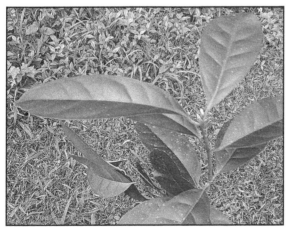

Ix tuc'ulil holds magical powers for the Maya because of its unique ability to cure sadness and relieve stress. The leaves are used as a bath to help with psychological problems.

Jesus Christ fern

Jesus Christ fern is a small fern with compound leaves divided three times. At each level the stems are alternate and are widest near the base, narrow at the tip. It has the unique property of being able to ressurect itself. If pulled up by its roots, the Jesus Christ fern might dry up, but once put in water, the fern will unfurl as when the leaves first unfurled.

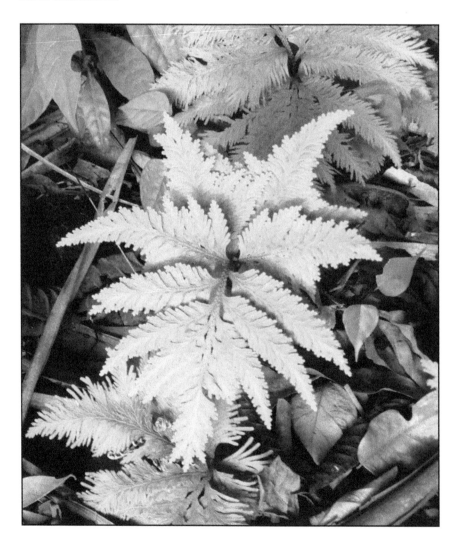

For prophetic dreams, put three Jesus Christ ferns, roots and all, in a glass of water and put it under your bed.

ko'mo' che'

Ko'mo' che' is a vine with narrow leaves with long pointed ends. The small yellow and red flowers grow underneath the leaves on the same stems.

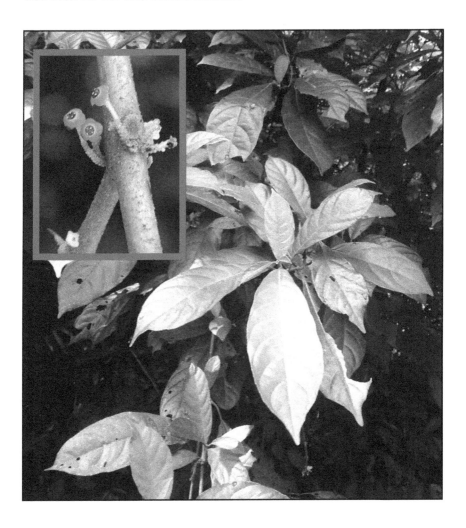

Ko'mo' che' is used for arthritis or rheumatism. Leaves and vine can be boiled and placed on the affected area. Tea made from ko'mo' che' leaves is good for bellyaches. Bathing with ko'mo'che leaves is helpful in the removal of ticks and lice. Ko'mo' che' tea is good for leishmaniasis and as an insect repellent. Washing with the tea removes swelling.

lengua de vaca, cow's tongue, hierba martina

Lengua de vaca grows as stiff stems (1 m long) with opposite yellowish-green narrow leaves with prominent veins ending in jagged edges. Clusters of small white flowers grow on separate stems from the leaves.

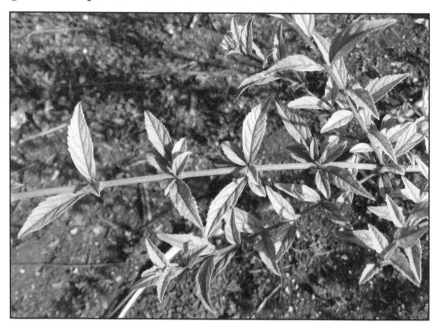

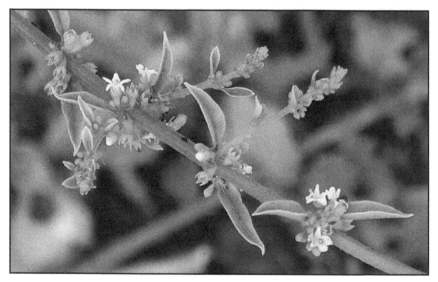

Lengua de vaca is used for de-worming and digestive problems, such as bellyache.

pasmo

Pasmo is a small plant with small pointed leaves with jagged edges. The fruits are small oblong balls, each on their own stem, which originates from the node of a leaf.

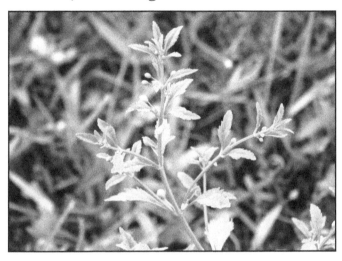

Tea from pasmo leaves is used to treat thickening of the blood.

pita haya

Pita haya is a cactus that grows on trees. The succulent leaves (3 cm wide) are smooth with spikes on the edges.

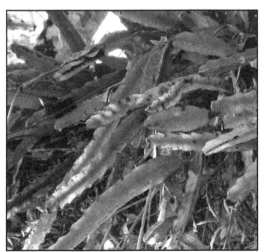 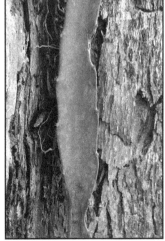

The inside of pita haya leaves is used as a hair conditioner.

policacia, colocho, lo'lo'och

Policacia grows into a large bush (3m high). The opposite leaves are divided into four to six round leaflets in a circle at the ends of stems. The leaflets have variable numbers of lobes with white on the zigzagged edges. Each vein in the leaflets ends in a tiny point.

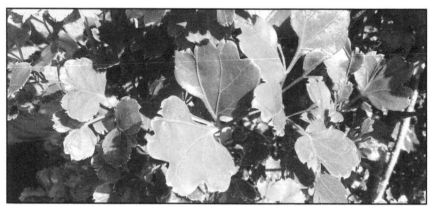

Policacia is good for labor pains. Boil one handful of leaves and drink it as a tea. It releases the pain. It is also good for premature contractions to hold the baby so that it stays in place.

tibush

Tibush is a grass that grows near the sea. The long (1 m) narrow leaves are green at first and then turn light brown, sometimes splitting near the top into several small leaves.

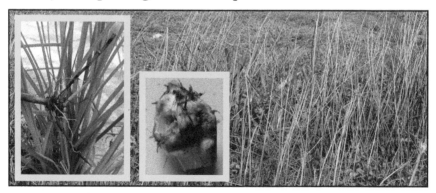

The tibush root is used to guard against evil spirits. A skull shape is carved from the root to make a bracelet for babies in red cloth. Extract the oil from the root and put on chakra sites to keep away evil spirits.

yax le'e

Yaxle'e grows as a bush with opposite large leaves (23 cm) that are shiny, grayish green, opposite, and triangular with pointed tips, rounded bases and jagged edges. The flowers are in clusters of many tubules at the ends of branched stems, opening to display fine hairs around the ends of the tubes.

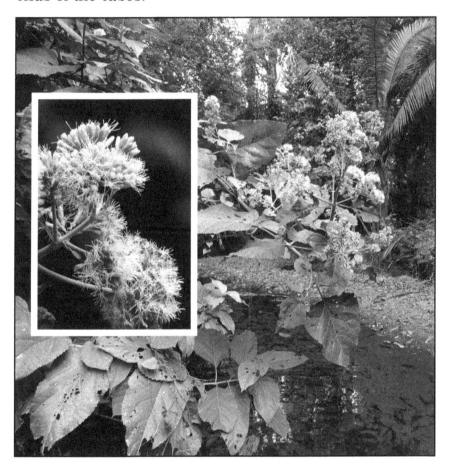

This is the one my uncle told me to use above all others, as it is the father of all herbs. It is good especially for cough, cold, fever, rheumatism, arthritis, inflammation, and pain. He used it for many pains in tincture or ointment and in holistic baths.

My Hopes for the Future

I increasingly see Mayan culture being left behind as we grow in a globalized world. Mayan customs are being lost to a monoculture, a culture that is being shaped by organized religion, modern technology and dominating westernized cultures. With every generation, fewer and fewer villages and peoples hold on to their heritage with a tight grasp.

My grandfather Juan Pasqual Mesh, was a snake doctor, a great healer in my village. That is why my mother knew a lot of plants, knowledge that she got from her father. But when we were growing up, he was not practicing the medicine anymore because he changed religion from Catholic to Pentecostal. He refused to practice herbal medicine because they told him it was bad. My mother used to tell us about him, saying that he dosed her with some type of powder made from some part of a poisonous snake to immunize her against poisonous snake bites. If a poisonous snake should bite her, it will do her no harm. But we never asked him what type of snake, what part of the snake, when to do it. That knowledge is now lost because his new religion made him think it was evil, so he did not pass along the knowledge. That is something very sad for us. We don't want that to happen anymore. Why would we allow others to come and tell us our knowledge is wrong?

Belize is a country rooted in Mayan history. It is a dream of mine, an attainable dream, that Belizeans and other Central Americans living in an area with a rich Mayan past will hold a respect for their country's sacred history. We have done a good job preserving many of the caves, what is believed to be the underworld, now if we can only do the same with the jungle, and the wild plants.

With a respect for plant life and herbal remedies will come a sense of reverence for the land and forests the plant life is born into. I hope to see more jungles preserved and awareness raised about the specific medicinal and edible qualities to both domesticated and wild plants. Ancient Maya knew their environment well, to the point that they could walk into the forest and gather specific plants for specific healings and meals. They had a connection with nature that few societies still hold. As they ate the natural foods they stayed healthier because the plants are medicine, too.

The path I see many societies going down is not one that is in conjunction with the health and good of the earth. We are losing respect for the earth and putting dependence on man-made goods. Our neighboring forests in Belize hold the answer to many illnesses and cancers. If we continue to degrade the earth, and lose the profound respect ancient Maya previously held for Mother Nature we will lose many of nature's healing powers. I can only hope future generations will come to know their land in the same way. The currrent Maya must find a way in which they can embrace their traditional beliefs and cultural heritage while incorporating modern living.

I am forever indebted to my village of San Antonio, a village that continues to hold on to their traditions and cultural heritage. My father was very intent on practicing Mayan religious ceremonies. I grew up seeing his dedication and the dedication of other family members. My great-uncle practiced herbal healings and my mother also held a deep knowledge of the healing power of plants and prayer.

Through this book, I have hoped to instill a sense of my passion for my culture into you, the reader. If there is the possibility that you can gain a sense of appreciation for Mayan heritage, and catch a glimpse of this rich culture through my eyes, I will be forever grateful. Please, do not let your understanding stop at the close of this book, but pass on your understanding of Mayan healing, herbal power, and the importance of keeping culture in the family.

Aurora Saqui

References

Balick, M.J., M.H. Nee, D.E. Atha. 2000. Checklist of Vascular Plants of Belize. *Memoirs of the New York Botanical Gardens*, 85: 1-246.

Kew. *Kew Herbarium Catalogue* <apps.kew.org/herbcat/navigator.do>.

Mabberley, D. J. 1987. *The Plant Book. A Portable Dictionary of the Higher Plants.* Cambridge UK: Cambridge University Press.

Missouri Botanical Gardens. *Tropicos* <tropicos.org>.

New York Botanical Garden. *Ethnobotany and Floristics of Belize Project* <sciweb.nybg.org/science2/hcol/beli/index.asp.html>.

New York Botanical Garden, International Plant Center. *The C.V. Star Virtual Herbarium* <sciweb.nybg.org/Science2/vii2.asp>.

Rietsema Jacob, D. Beveridge. 2009. *The Plants of Caye Caulker.* Caye Caulker, Belize: *Produccciones de la Hamaca.*

Royal Botanic Gardens, Kew and Missouri Botanical Garden. *The Plant List: A Working list of All Plants* <theplantlist.org>.

Index

A

a'bül 128
a'bül po'ok'oc 127
Acacia cornigera 39, 42
acaliptus 37, 39, 140
Acalypha arvensis 39, 43
aceite ko'och 118
Adiantum concinnum 40, 44
adormidilla 94
AIDS vi, 19, 57, 97, 117
alambre 90
albahaca 98
alepa 10, 21, 39, 82
allergies vi, 19
allspice 26, 35, 39, 104
aloe 23, 28, 30, 39, 45
Aloe vera 39, 45
Amaranthus dubius 39, 46
Anacardium occidentale 39, 47
Ananas comosus 41, 48
anemia vi, 19
angel's trumpet 20, 39, 53
anger vi, 20
anjus a'ck 51
Annona muricata 41, 49
Anthurium schlechtendalii 41
apasote 36, 39, 73
arbol de pito 75
Aristolochia trilobata 39, 51
arthritis vi, 20, 24
asthma vi, 20
athlete's foot vi, 20
Attalea cohune 39, 52
avocado 11, 12, 20, 21, 24, 29, 39, 100

B

baalche ha' 17
bad luck vi, 21
bad spirits vi, 21
balance vi, 21
basil 10, 15, 25, 26, 27, 31, 35, 36, 39, 98
basket tie-tie 22, 39, 70
bath 10, 11
baths 10

bayal 70
bay cedar 32, 39, 79
bayel 70
beef worm vi, 21
behavior vi, 21
behavior problems 21
beneno xut 15, 39, 141
bird pepper 33, 39, 56
birth 31
bleeding vi, 21
blood pressure vi, 22
blood purifier vi, 22
bob 39, 142
bok 15, 20
bot fly vi, 21
breast feeding 22
brittle maidenhair fern 44
broom palm 67
Brugmansia suaveolens 39, 53
bucut 32, 37, 39, 58
bullhorn 42
burns vi, 23
burrowing form of bot fly 21
Bursera simaruba 40, 54
buttonwood 107
Byrsonima crassifolia 39, 55

C

cacao 10, 14-18, 22, 25, 29, 33, 39, 135
calaloo 46
calawala 29, 39, 102, 143
callaloo 25, 39, 46
campana top' 53
cancer vi, 23, 43
cancer herb 35, 39, 43
candle bush 122
can'il 20
Capsicum frutescens 39, 56
Carica papaya 40, 57
cashew 37, 39, 47
Cassia grandis 39, 58
castor bean 118
castor oil plant 28, 30, 32, 37, 39, 118

cat's tongue 114
cecropia 19, 22, 26, 30, 35, 39,
    59, 80
Cecropia peltata 39, 59
cedar 21, 26, 32, 39, 60, 79
Cedrela odorata 39, 60
cedro 60
ceiba 11, 14, 39, 61
Ceiba pentandra 39, 61
cha'al che' 24, 31, 32, 39, 111
chaca' 54
chatchi 71
chate 71
chaya 18, 19, 31, 39, 63
chi' 55
chichibeh 123
chicle 32, 37, 39, 93
chiclera 32, 58
chili pepper 56
chillon che' 76
cilantro simaron 74
Citrus aurantifolia 40, 62
Cnidoscolus chayamansa 39, 63
Cochlospermum vitifolium 41, 64
cockspur 11, 20, 32, 39, 42
coco 65
cocoa 135
coconut 15, 38, 39, 65
Cocos nucifera 39, 65
cohune palm 18, 39, 52
cojoton 132
cola de mico 39, 92, 102,143
cold vi, 24
colocho 151
common rue 119
contraception vi, 24
contribo 19, 27, 30, 36, 39, 51
copal 12, 13, 14, 17, 21, 25, 28,
    29, 35, 39, 42, 115, 133
corazon 39, 144
corbata 50
cordoncillo 39, 107
corn 9, 14, 22, 33, 36, 39, 82, 138
corremiento 90
costa plant 66
Costus pulverulentu 41
cot-acam 130

cotton 12, 13, 24, 30, 34, 39, 41,
    61, 64, 78
cotton tree 61
cough 12, 24, 34
cough bush 111
cough syrup 12, 20, 34, 49,100,
    130,156
cowfoot 30, 31, 34, 35, 36, 39,
    105, 106, 107
cow's tongue 150
craboo 39, 55
croton 133
Cryosophila stauracantha 40, 67
crystal 5, 6, 7, 14
culantrillo 72
culantro 27, 34, 36, 39, 74
cupping 12
cure-for-all 112
Cyathea myosuroides 41, 68
Cymbopogon citratus 40, 69

D
datura 53
dehydration vi, 25
delivery vii, 31
depression vi, 25
Desmoncus orthacanthos 39, 70
diabetes vi, 26
Dialium guianense 40
diarrhea 7, 26, 47, 55, 79, 87,
    94, 104, 116
Dicranopteris pectinata 41, 72
digestion 26
doncella 27
duck flower 51
dysentery bark 124
Dysphania ambrosioides 39, 73

E
ears vi, 27, 138
ehimbre 139
ensalmo 16, 36
epazote 73
Eryngium foetidum 39, 74
Erythrina folkersii 41, 75
escoba 67
Eugenia ibarrae 41, 76
evil eye 27, 99, 103

eyes 27, 32, 56

F
fern 21, 29, 31, 39, 40, 41, 44,
        68, 72, 90, 91, 92, 129
fern hetero 39, 90
fern venus 29, 40, 91
fever vi, 28
flor de pato 51
flu vi, 24
frijolillo 17, 20, 24, 28, 40, 122
fungus vi, 20

G
Garcia sisters x
sisters viii, 1
gastritis 27, 85
gel 13
general health vi, 28
ginger 24, 26, 36, 40, 139
give-and-take palm 40, 67
Gliricidia sepium 40, 77
glue tree 40
golden plum 37, 40, 127
good luck charms 14
Gossypium hirsutum 39, 78
guanábana 49
guava 7, 26, 31, 33, 37, 40, 116
Guazuma ulmifolia 39, 79
gumbolimbo 15, 32, 33, 35, 36,
        40, 54
guyaba 116

H
hagan u yool 36
hair 29
hakil olal 36
hamans 22, 36, 40, 132
Hamelia patens 41, 80
harry tom 103
headache vi, 29
helecho 68
hepatitis vi, 30
hibiscus 21, 25, 29, 40, 81
Hibiscus rosa-sinensis 40, 81
hierba buena 40, 113
hierba del cancer 43
hierba de piojillo 112
hierba martina 149

hierba preniada 144
higuerilla 118
hog plum 7, 19, 23, 28, 32,37,
        40, 129
horse balls 131
horse bush 40, 145
hot flashes vii, 31
ho'tz 40, 145
huevo de caballo 131
huhub 129

I
Immune System vi, 30
Incense 12
Indian almond 132
indigestion 7, 26, 27, 51, 117
infertility vi, 30
inflammation vii, 30
insect repellent 15
Ipomoea sp 39
ironwood 40, 71
ix bra' haj 121
ix calalo 46
ix cat 40, 146
ix cha'al che' 111
ix ka'nan 80
ix mu'tz 94
ix placan 99
ix shim 138
ix tabay 114
ix tuc'ulil 10, 25, 31, 34, 35, 40,
        147
ix yamor 95

J
jackass bitters 15, 21, 26, 31,
        32, 33, 40, 97
jaundice vi, 30
Jesus Christ fern 148
jocote 128
Justicia breviflora 41, 83

K
kach okpitch 20, 40, 44
kakaltun 98
Kalanchoe pinnata 41, 84
kekeltun 98
keletus 140
k'eletush 140

k'le'tux 140
ko'mo' che' 15, 20, 21, 30-32,
        34, 40, 149
ko'och 28,118
ku' che 60
ku' ku' 134

L
lantana 85
Lantana camara 41, 85
Lantana involucrata 41
laxative vii, 30
lemongrass 12, 28, 40, 69
lengua de vaca 40, 150
Licania platypus 40, 87
life everlasting 84
lime 11, 18, 21, 24, 32, 33, 35,
        40, 62
limon 62
Lippia alba 41, 88
Lippia graveolens 41, 89
lo'lo'och 150
Lygodium heterodoxum 40, 90
Lygodium venustum 40, 91

M
madre cacao 10, 40, 77
maize 138
mallard stone 27, 36, 40, 103
malo de ojo 6, 27
malva 17, 29, 36, 40, 123
ma'mu'kal 15, 34, 40, 112
Mangifera indica 40, 92
mango 12, 23, 28, 40, 92
Manilkara zapota 39, 93
mano de lagarto 97
maranion 47
mash ik 56
massage 15
may plum 33, 37, 40, 128
menopause vii, 31
menstruation 31
Mexican oregano 89
migraine vi, 29
miis 67
mimosa 95
Mimosa pudica 41, 94
Momordica charantia 41, 95

monkey apple 26, 30, 40, 87
Morinda citrifolia 40, 96
Moses-in-the-boat 135
moses-in-the-cradle 33, 40
mosote 7, 36, 40, 114
mother-in-law tongue 40, 120
mumps vii, 31
mun nal 138
mun nil 138
muscle cramps vii, 31
muscle weakness vii, 31
mutazai 28, 40, 101

N
naba kuuk 26, 31,104
nance 55
na' suuon 97
negrito 27, 40, 124
Neurolaena lobata 40, 97
noni 19, 26, 28, 40, 96
nopal 99
nuuk lea' 89
nuuk suun 97

O
obel 107
Ocimum basilicum 39, 98
oil 15
ointment 15
oon 101
Opuntia cochenillifera 41, 99
oregano 86
ore'go 88
ore'go ich che' 85

P
pain vii, 31
palo de hombre 19, 22, 25, 27,
        28, 30, 31, 36, 37, 40, 117
palo de lacandon 71
Panti, Elijio ii, viii, ix, 2, 3, 4,
        5, 8
papaya 19, 22, 26, 30, 40, 57
paralysis vii, 31
pasmo 11, 41, 85, 151
patez 16, 35
p'a tzi'min 131
pear 101
pech ma'am 115

peltatum piper 19, 41, 105
Persea americana 31
pheasant tail 10, 17, 41, 50
philodendron 21, 28, 41, 101
Philodendron hederaceum 40, 101
Philodendron sp. 41, 101
Phlebodium decumanum 39, 102
Phyllanthus amarus 40, 103
pi' che' 83
pik 11
Pimenta dioica 39, 104
pimienta gorda 104
piña 48
pineapple 41, 48
pinkroot 126
piper 10, 11, 15-17, 20, 25, 29, 30, 31, 33-35, 41, 106-110
Piper auritum 39, 106
Piper jacquemontianum 39, 107
Piper peltatum 41, 105
Piper pseudolindenii 41
Piper sp. 41, 108-110
pirish 11
piss-a-bed 19, 26, 30, 35, 41, 121
pita haya 29, 41, 151
pito 35, 41, 75
pito coral tree 75
pitz 78
pixoy 79
Pluchea carolinensis 39, 111
policacia 31, 32, 41, 152
polished maidenhair fern 44
polly redhead 15, 19, 21, 26, 27, 30, 33, 36, 37, 41, 80
pom 12, 115
po'ok'oc 129
Porophyllum punctatum 40
Portulaca oleracea 40, 113
poultice 16
powder 16
prayers 16
pregnancy vii, 31
prickly pear 29, 41, 99
Priva lappulacea 40, 114
protection iv, vii, 32
Protium copal 39, 115

Psidium guajava 40, 116
p'tah 116
pu' chuch 107
punse 11
purge vii, 32
put' 57

Q
Quassia amara 40, 117
qui cun naj 14

R
rabbit's paw 41, 125
red copal 133
red incense 32, 33, 41, 133
red polywood 80
rheumatism vi, 20
Ricinus communis 39, 118
rudah 10, 15, 25, 31, 41, 119
Ruta chalepensis 41, 119

S
sacate' limon 69
sansapote 87
Sansevieria hyacinthoides 40, 120
santa maria 111
sapodilla 93
sa' wan 137
Senna alata 41, 121
Senna occidentalis 40, 122
sensitive plant 33, 41, 94
Sida acuta 40, 124
siempreviva 30, 31, 41, 84
Simarouba glauca 40, 124
sink-and-bible 45
skin lesions vii, 32
skunk root 83
sleep vii, 33
small oregano 27, 36, 37, 41, 88
smudge 17, 25, 28, 29, 35, 115
snakebite vii, 34
sore throat vii, 34
sorosi 18, 22, 23, 25, 31, 41, 95
soursop 12, 23, 36, 41, 49
Spanish elder 107
Sphagneticola trilobata 41, 125
spiderwort 135
Spigelia anthelmia 41, 126
Spondias mombin 40, 127

Spondias purpurea 40, 128
Spondias radlkoferi 40, 129
sprains vii, 34
squirrel's tail 112
Stachytarpheta cayennensis 41, 130
staircase plant 27, 32, 41, 66
Stemmadenia donnell-smithii 40, 131
stinking toe 58
stomach 34
stomach ulcers vii, 34
stone breaker 103
stress vii, 34
stroke vii, 34
subin 42
succotz 87

T
tah tai'i 112
tapaculo 79
Terminalia catappa 40, 132
Tetragastris panamensis 41, 133
Theobroma cacao 39, 134
thick oregano 12, 27, 30, 31, 37, 41, 89
thorn vii, 35
tibush 41, 152
tiger fern 31, 41, 72
tincture 17
tobacco 35
tobacco smoking addiction 35
tonic 18
tonsilitis vii, 34
toothache vii, 35
tourist tree 54
Tradescantia spathacea 40, 135
trauma vii, 35
tree fern 41, 68
tres puntas 97
trumpet tree 59
tucul 26
tuculil 26
tulipan 81
tumor vii, 35
tumun 78
tuz 52

twelve o'clock 94
tzak pol 29

U
ujanal atu'rich 125
ulcers 34
u'moch atu'rich 125
urinary problems vii, 35

V
verbena 12, 29, 41, 130
verdolaga 113
vervain 130
vision 36
Vitex gaumeri 41, 136
Vochysia hondurensis 41, 137

W
wanabe 49
warumo 59
weight reduction vii, 36
white mahogany 137
wild berry 41, 76
wild cilantro 74
wild cotton 30, 41, 64
wild cucumber 145
wild grape 20, 41, 86
wild oregano 11, 26, 27, 41, 85
wild spinach 46
wild tamarin 71
wire wisk 90
worm bush 21, 41, 126
worms vii, 36
wound healing vii, 37

X
xhi'ic ku'tz 130

Y
ya' 93
yax le'e 5, 41, 153
yaxnik 32, 41, 136
yellow jaundice 30
yemeri 21, 32, 41, 137

Z
Zea mays 39, 138
Zingiber officinale 40, 139
zorillo macho 32, 33, 34, 35, 41, 83